# China's Livestock Revolution: Agribusiness and policy developments in the sheep meat industry

Dedicated to the girls:
Zoe, Sarah, Imogen, Eloise, Yudong and Yuxi

# China's Livestock Revolution: Agribusiness and policy developments in the sheep meat industry

**Scott Waldron**
**Colin Brown**
**John Longworth**
**Zhang Cungen**

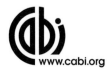

www.cabi.org

**CABI is a trading name of CAB International**

| | |
|---|---|
| CABI Head Office | CABI North American Office |
| Nosworthy Way | 875 Massachusetts Avenue |
| Wallingford | 7th Floor |
| Oxfordshire OX10 8DE | Cambridge, MA 02139 |
| UK | USA |
| Tel: +44 (0)1491 832111 | Tel: +1 617 395 4056 |
| Fax: +44 (0)1491 833508 | Fax: +1 617 354 6875 |
| E-mail: cabi@cabi.org | E-mail: cabi-nao@cabi.org |
| Website: www.cabi.org | |

A catalogue record for this book is available from the British Library, London, UK.

A catalogue record for this book is available from the Library of Congress, Washington, DC.

ISBN: 978 1 84593 246 6

Printed and bound in the UK from copy supplied by the editors by Athenaeum Press, Gateshead.

# Contents

**List of tables**

## List of boxes

## List of figures and maps

## List of images

# Preface

The international livestock revolution has received a level of attention in line with its profound worldwide implications. The Chinese livestock sector leads the revolution in terms of its aggregate size and growth rate. Like the livestock sectors of many other developing countries that have been swept up in the revolution, the Chinese livestock sector has also undergone dramatic structural change. Despite the enormous importance of the developments in China, it is difficult to obtain detailed information about what is going on in the Chinese livestock sector, especially in relation to the ruminant livestock industries. Given that the China Agricultural Economics Group of the University of Queensland has been researching the ruminant livestock sector in China for two decades, we felt that we could contribute to a better understanding of the international livestock revolution by providing a micro level study of a Chinese ruminant livestock industry.

Although the book focuses on the Chinese sheep meat industry, it draws heavily on associated research on other aspects of the Chinese livestock sector. The China Agricultural Economics Group has conducted major research projects on all aspects of the wool, beef and now sheep meat industries. The research has also addressed issues closely related to ruminant livestock industries such as rangeland degradation and minority nationalities. One of the guiding principles of this ongoing research has been to understand how development of the livestock sector can be harnessed to achieve widespread development of the rural sector. Prolonged periods of fieldwork for this research have been conducted in more than half the provinces in China and many of these areas have been visited several times over the last 20 years.

This long term research in a range of industries and areas provides a valuable background against which to analyse what is happening in the Chinese sheep meat industry. It has enabled the authors to use the sheep meat case study to illustrate many broader trends and insights that apply more generally to the Chinese livestock sector, especially the ruminant livestock part of that sector.

Developments in the Chinese ruminant livestock industries over this period have been marked by both continuity and change. For example, the vertically integrated 'dragon head' enterprises established to lead the modernization of the sector, bear many resemblances and perform similar industry functions to the State agencies that they have replaced, though under different ownership structures. Whilst production and marketing systems are still dominated by 'the multitude' of small, semi-subsistence households, the more progressive or better connected households have become larger and more specialized. Most Chinese still buy their food from wet markets but wealthier urban residents can now purchase from chains of supermarkets and franchise restaurants. An enormous hierarchy of Party, state and quasi state officials still attempts to oversee, plan and influence industry participants and outcomes, with varying degrees of success. Against this background, many industry participants, researchers and extension agents in China are looking for ways to increase the competitiveness of the livestock industries and to orient them toward broader societal objectives.

A large proportion of the information in this book came first hand from these industry participants. The spirit of cooperation and the frank and open discussions that provided this information is gratefully acknowledged. Hopefully this book will go some way toward repaying these industry people by contributing to the continued healthy development of the Chinese livestock sector and helping the world understand it better.

As the Chinese and international livestock industries become more enmeshed, detailed and accurate information about developments in China will become increasingly crucial. Policy makers and industry leaders in the livestock sectors of other countries are recognizing the need to understand and communicate with counterparts in China. Meat and Livestock Australia is a leader in this regard. As part of its activities in China, in 2003 Meat and Livestock Australia commissioned the China Agricultural Economics Group to conduct research and write a report on 'An Analysis of agribusiness and policy developments in China's sheep meat industry of relevance to the Australian industry'. This project provided the funding and impetus to make this book possible. Thus, we would like to thank Meat and Livestock Australia for the resources and willingness to genuinely understand the market in which it operates. In particular we would like to thank Tim Kelf, Sylvia Athas and Elisa Tseng for close support and feedback throughout the project and Leith Tilley for valuable comments and information during the preparation of this book. We would also like to thank Meat and Livestock Australia and the Australian Centre for International Agricultural Research for funding other related China Agricultural Economics Group research projects in China.

The detailed research upon which this book is based was a team effort involving many people and the authors would like to thank these professional colleagues for their contributions. Much of the information – both primary and secondary – was collected by researchers from the Institute of Agricultural Economics of the Chinese Academy of Agricultural Sciences, including Deng Rong, Xiong Cunkai, Wang Xiangyang and Liu Fang. The research support and facilities of the Institute of Agricultural Economics were also very much appreciated. Lu Xiaoping from the Ministry of Agriculture helped in his usual friendly and efficient way to facilitate field work. Zhao Yutian from the Research Centre for the Rural Economy within the Ministry of Agriculture attended fieldwork for a concurrent wool project and for certain periods of the sheep meat project. His expertise and interest in the sheep industry was of considerable benefit to the project. Zheng Shaofeng from the Northwest Scientech University of Agriculture and Forestry contributed interesting data and analysis on household livestock production that appears in Chapter 3. Ian Auldist provided well grounded knowledge from Chifeng.

In Brisbane, the School of Natural and Rural Systems Management at the University of Queensland and many of its staff provided an environment conducive to productive research. Stephanie Cash demonstrated amazing skills to produce a sophisticated report on which this book is based. Richard Hudson and his team at Sunset Digital provided timely and meticulous setting services for the production of this book. Finally, we would like to thank CAB International for adding this book to their unsurpassed list of titles in the field of agriculture and for the support to get the book to press.

Although this book is the result of a large team effort, responsibility for any errors or misinterpretations remains with the authors. While this book seeks to provide a detailed account of the Chinese sheep meat industry and the drivers of change, it is an analysis of a highly dynamic industry. All information in the book should therefore be updated and verified before being used for commercial purposes.

A final note on conventions: there are no acronyms used in this book and only two uniquely Chinese units are mentioned. The Chinese currency renminbi is abbreviated as 'Rmb' and at the time of the research there was approximately Rmb8.3 to the United States dollar. The Chinese unit of land area is 'mu' and there is 15 mu to the hectare. The title 'Inner Mongolia' abbreviates 'Inner Mongolia Autonomous Region' while 'Xinjiang' abbreviates 'Xinjiang Uygur Autonomous Region'.

Scott Waldron
Colin Brown
John Longworth
Zhang Cungen

June 2006

*China's Livestock Revolution*

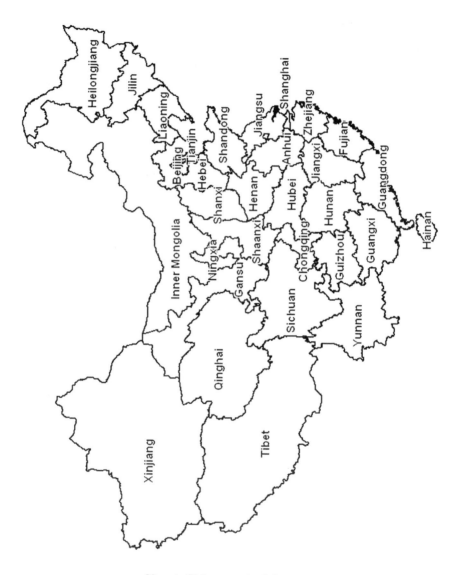

**Map 1. China provincial map.**

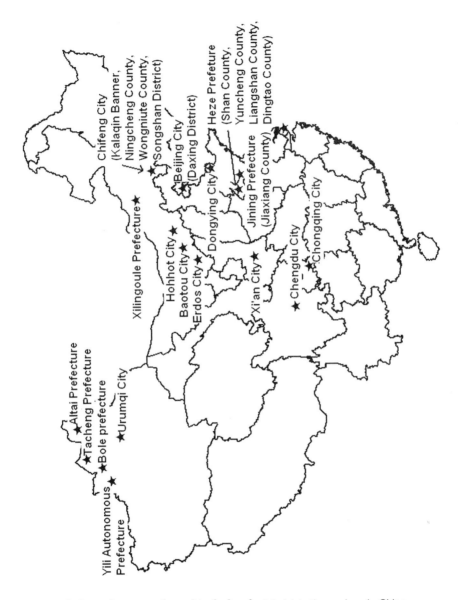

**Map 2. Selected areas referred to in book.** Administrative regions in China are organized into a defined hierarchy. For the purposes of this map, the centre is at the highest level, followed by provinces and autonomous regions (see Map 1, and the province level cities of Beijing, Shanghai and Chongqing in this Map 2), the capital cities of provinces and autonomous regions (Xi'an, Chengdu, Hohhot, Urumqi), prefectures and their equivalents (Chifeng, Xilingoule, Baotou, Heze, Jining, Dongying, Yili, Bole, Tacheng, Altai), city districts (Daxing) followed by counties and their equivalents (Kalaqin, Ningcheng, Wongniute, Songshan, Shan, Yuncheng, Liangshan, Dingtao and Jiaxiang).

# 1
# China and the international livestock revolution

The world is in the midst of what has been dubbed a 'livestock revolution' with far reaching implications for human health, development, the environment and trade (Delgado *et al.*, 1999). China is at the forefront of this revolution. Developments in China's livestock sector will impact on the flows of food, feed and livestock products on an international level (Simpson *et al.*, 1994; Simpson, 2003; Nin *et al.*, 2004; Zhou and Tian, 2005). Within China, the livestock sector has been an engine of growth in the broader agricultural sector, and the economic 'pillar' of many underdeveloped parts of China. Despite its importance, few English language studies examine the intricacies of China's livestock revolution – how real it is, what drives it, how it is reflected in agribusiness structures, and its implications. This book seeks to do so through the window of China's emerging sheep meat industry.

## 1.1 China's role in the international livestock revolution

The absolute increase in the market value of global meat and milk production between the early 1970s and the mid 1990s was more than double the increase in cereals production brought about by the better known 'green revolution' (Delgado *et al.*, 1999). Like the green revolution, the so called 'livestock revolution' has taken place in the developing world. Whereas the production and consumption of livestock products has stalled in the developed world, both have taken off in the developing world. With consumption levels of meat still one third lower than those of the developed countries, the rapid expansion of the livestock sector in the developing world could be expected to continue for some time.

China is the major player in the international livestock sector in all but a few industries.[1] Figure 1.1 shows the annual growth rates in meat production (including pork, poultry, beef, sheep meat and goat meat) for selected country

---

1. For example, India is much more important than China in the dairy industry.

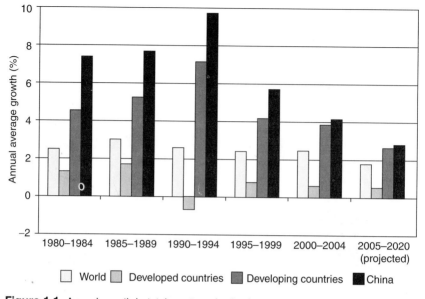

**Figure 1.1.** Annual growth in total meat production by country groupings, 1980 to 2020. *Source*: Food and Agriculture Organization (last accessed August 2005).

groupings between 1980 and 2004.[2] While average growth rates in meat production over this period were around 3% for the world as a whole, there was considerable variation across countries. Meat production in developed countries grew by only 1%, compared with 5% in developing countries and 7% in China. Indeed, the high growth rate and the large size of the industry in China had a major impact on the figures for the 'world' and 'developing countries' categories which would be both scaled back by at least 1% if China was excluded. Delgado *et al.* (1999) project that the differentials will diminish into the longer term future (to 2020) but that China will still sustain higher growth than the other regions.

Although Figure 1.2 does not reflect China's relatively modest international trade flows in livestock and meat products, or the relatively low value of

---

2. Data in this section are derived from the FAOSTAT database (Food and Agriculture Organization, accessed August 2005) except for projections to 2020 which are drawn from Delgado *et al.* (1999). The data has made some allowances for the inaccuracies of Chinese official data. Fuller *et al.* (2000) state that from 1984 to 1994, Food and Agriculture Organization statistics for Chinese meat production lie 'above or less than' 15% below the numbers of the Chinese State Statistical Bureau, except for beef production, which lies 10% to 25% below official Chinese figures. However, the differences between Food and Agriculture Organization and Chinese official statistics are now negligible. Delgado *et al.* (1999) claim that they use conservative estimates of Chinese data for their projections, and that even a radical downsizing of the Chinese data does not dramatically alter the conclusions. The 2004 FAOSTAT data was provisional and was not compared with the official Chinese data. This is because in early 2006 when this book was being completed, the 2005 yearbooks which contain 2004 data had not been released. However, unpublished sources from the Chinese Ministry of Agriculture are used in some cases in this book for 2004 and 2005 data.

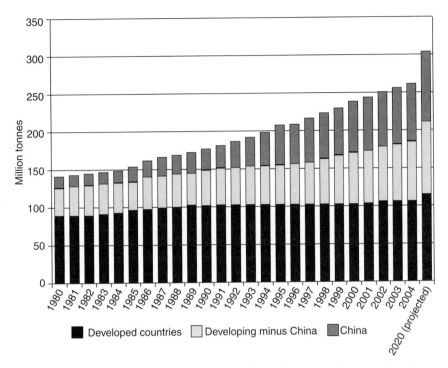

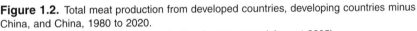

**Figure 1.2.** Total meat production from developed countries, developing countries minus China, and China, 1980 to 2020.
*Source*: Food and Agriculture Organization (last accessed August 2005).

production of the sector, it does show China's pre-eminent position in the international livestock sector in terms of production. China now accounts for nearly one third of world meat production and nearly one half of meat production in developing countries. Projections from Delgado *et al.* (1999) indicate that this dominance will be further consolidated in the future.

It should also be noted that the size of China's livestock industry is not just a function of its human demographics. Per capita meat production figures in Figure 1.3 demonstrate that levels in China were on par with those in developing countries as a whole in 1980, but by the mid 1990s had risen to above world levels. Delgado *et al.* (1999) forecast that per capita meat production in China will be two thirds as high as that in developed countries by 2020.

## 1.2 Understanding China's livestock revolution

Although aggregate statistics capture China's influential role in the international livestock sector, they represent just the tip of the iceberg. That is, they are the visible outcomes of more deep rooted forces. This book aims to examine the livestock sector in much greater detail and depth in the manner outlined in Figure 1.4.

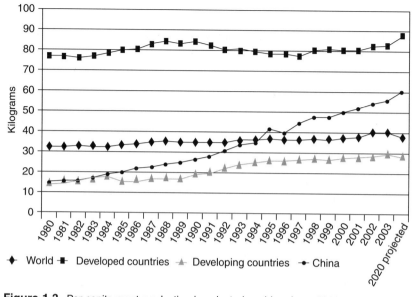

**Figure 1.3.** Per capita meat production in selected world regions, 1980 to 2020. *Source*: Food and Agriculture Organization (last accessed August 2005).

The organization of the book enables a progression from a macro level to micro level analysis. Aggregate statistics are the broadest indicators of industry developments and so are a widely used entry point for understanding the livestock sector. The popular usage of macro statistics warrants a critical analysis of their strengths, limitations and how they can be analysed and interpreted and this is covered in Chapters 2 and 3.

The second level of analysis and second part of the book addresses the underlying drivers behind the trends and patterns observed in the aggregate statistics. Market drivers are discussed in Chapter 3 (which include the presentation of market related statistics), while institutional drivers are examined in Chapter 4 and policy drivers in Chapter 5. These drivers lie behind the industry developments reflected in the statistical indicators. However, the relationship is not unidimensional as the statistics are an important input into policy and commercial decisions.

The third and most detailed level of analysis is conducted on industry and agribusiness systems. These are organized in line with the flow of commodities along the supply chain, from sheep breeding, production and marketing (Chapter 6) to sheep meat production and marketing (Chapter 7). Industry drivers (discussed in Chapters 3, 4 and 5) forge industry and agribusiness structures (Chapters 6 and 7) but the relationship is also two way. That is, the nature of the industry structures affect policy making and institutional structures governing the industry. Before turning attention to these detailed issues and chapters, the discussion below briefly sets out the themes to be analysed.

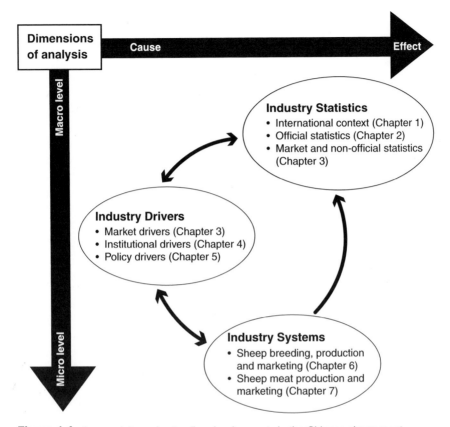

**Figure 1.4.** Approach to understanding developments in the Chinese sheep meat industry.

### 1.2.1 Statistical issues

The accuracy of Chinese livestock statistics has been and remains a major concern (United States Department of Agriculture, 1998; Fuller *et al.*, 2000; Ke, 2001). Statistical collection has been extremely difficult in China since decollectivization and economic liberalization that began in 1979. Hundreds of millions of households in China raise livestock on a very low scale of production, often in the range of a few head per household. Supply chains are dominated by hundreds of thousands of small traders and processors, rather than centralized slaughter and auction systems that facilitate statistical collection in developed countries. The bottom up reporting system (from village up to central level) gives scope for tens of thousands of officials to over report, which they do to fill higher level administrative, production oriented, decrees and to increase their chances of promotion.

Aware of the inaccuracies, China conducted a National Agricultural Census in 1997. Results from the census led to massive downward revisions of meat production for 1996 by 20%. Beef was revised most drastically by 28%, followed by sheep and goat meat by 27.8% (United States Department of Agriculture, 1998). Fuller *et al.* (2000) suggest that actual pork production levels may be 39% lower, while actual poultry production could be 70% lower than official National Bureau of Statistics statistics. They argue that average annual growth rates for beef, pork, and poultry production are at least 5% below the numbers implied by published data sources, and that livestock inventory and slaughter numbers may be greatly overstated.

The most obvious discrepancy in the official Chinese livestock statistics is that livestock production greatly exceeded consumption and does not reconcile with net trade volumes (Ke, 2001). In addition to the problems of overstated production, the discrepancy reflects problems in accurately identifying consumption. Official consumption data does not take into account 'out of home' consumption (estimated to be one third of consumption in urban areas), or the 'floating population' of rural people working in cities (estimated to be between 100 million and 130 million people). Meat consumption (bone out) and meat production (bone in) are also not compared on an equivalent basis. For these reasons, Ke (2001) estimates that actual meat consumption figures may have been under reported by 40 to 50%.

In light of the serious flaws in the reporting of official livestock statistics in China, a critical approach to interpretation of the statistics is required. Apart from reporting these statistics, Chapter 2 provides an examination of the way by which official livestock statistics are derived and highlights the systematic biases that arise. Although it is beyond the scope of this book to collate alternative figures to the official ones, the analyses reported in Chapters 2 and 3 add value to the official statistics by incorporating non official or more disaggregated data, alternative technical parameters and alternative methodologies. Statistical discrepancies and issues are addressed in more detail in Chapter 2.

### 1.2.2 Drivers of China's livestock revolution

In accessing the statistical accuracy and growth of the Chinese livestock sector, questions arise as to what is driving the growth. Delgado *et al.* (1999) state explicitly – and most other studies assume implicitly – that the international livestock revolution is market driven, and is different in this regard to the green revolution which was supply driven. Market drivers include population growth, rising incomes, urbanization, and consumer preferences shifting toward animal products and proteins. Furthermore, the increasingly liberalized market environment means that livestock producers and other industry actors are increasingly able to respond to these consumer demands. The market – or demand-pull – drivers will continue to drive growth and development of the livestock sector into the longer term future, and are examined in detail in Chapter 3.

However, one of the distinguishing features of the livestock sector in China is that non market forces have also been a major driver of change. In particular, powerful state structures have the capacity to fast track the development of industries in China and have provided enormous support and intervention in the production and processing sides of the industry. These policy-push drivers have been exerted strongly in a range of new livestock industries, including beef, dairy and – as discussed in Chapters 4 and 5 – sheep meat. The policy push notionally is designed to pre-empt market signals, to be market complying and ultimately phased out and to be overtaken by longer term market drivers.

The interaction between market-pull and policy-push drivers is crucial to understanding both the growth – the expansion of output – and the development – which includes moving up value chains in a sustainable manner – of Chinese livestock industries. Industry policies are often aimed at kick-starting industry growth, industry modernization and achieving various strategic and social objectives.[3] Institutions and policies are also important in the longer term development of the livestock sector. Market services (such as standards, grading and information) and production services (such as extension and local group formation) forge the environment in which livestock industries and markets operate, and change incentives for industry participants. Thus any analysis of developments in the Chinese livestock sector requires a detailed treatment of policy and institutional forces.

### 1.2.3 Industry and agribusiness structures

Although the drivers mentioned above help forge the path for industry development, so too do the underlying structures of the industries. Appreciating industry structures in China's complex and fast changing agribusiness environment is no easy task and requires extensive primary fieldwork and data. The third level of analysis in the book (Chapters 6 and 7) investigates agribusiness changes in both sheep and sheep meat production and marketing.

Various themes emerge from the agribusiness analysis including the way by which industry stages and actors coordinate – or otherwise – to bring about rapid growth. The dominant feature of livestock industry structures in China is their small scale and fragmented nature, especially in livestock production and marketing. The very low scales of household livestock production systems pose technical and economic constraints on industry development, and challenges for extension, marketing, disease control and environmental activities. Similar issues arise in the slaughter, livestock marketing and meat marketing sectors that are dominated by households and private dealers. The way that these small scale

---

3. A major theme in the livestock revolution literature is that public policies and services need to be oriented in a way that will facilitate rural development broadly defined to include the interests of smallholders and their integration into markets, the environment and food safety (see Delgado *et al.*, 1999 and Waldron *et al.*, 2003).

and fragmented structures evolve through household specialization, cooperative activities and corporatization and how they are influenced by specific policies will be of major economic and social consequence.

Traditionally, agricultural policy in China has had a strong bias toward production. In the case of livestock, for example, breeding, feeding and veterinary activities have been a major focus of policy and through the extension system. More recently, the supply bias of policy has been extended to encouraging the formation of large (usually quasi state) enterprises to modernize both the provision of inputs (feed, genetics, veterinary products) and the marketing of farm outputs. These new agribusiness structures encourage integration across the various stages of production and marketing. Of course, as households are still by far the most important actors in the industries, an understanding of the manner in which households interface with these new structures (such as via contracts, associations and networks) is crucial.

An inter-related feature of Chinese livestock industries not reflected in the aggregate data is that the vast majority of livestock products in China are low quality and low value. This is a result of the alignment of the small scale of production and marketing structures with demand side factors including low average consumer incomes, the localized nature of consumption, and Chinese cooking and consumption practices. However, livestock officials and actors are now turning attention from quantity toward quality issues. The process of market segmentation into a variety of premium or non mass market segments is an especially important aspect of industry development.

## 1.3 The Chinese sheep meat industry as a case study

Developments in the Chinese livestock sector are analysed in this book through the window of the sheep meat industry. Apart from global interest in the industry itself, the sheep meat industry provides an excellent illustration of three sets of issues confronting anyone seeking an understanding of the Chinese livestock sector: namely the interpretation of statistics, industry drivers and agribusiness structures.

Sheep meat is one of a number of livestock industries in China to have emerged only in recent years. Indeed, while the sheep meat industry has grown substantially for two decades, it only began commercializing and orienting toward specialized sheep meat production and consumption in the mid to late 1990s. As such, the sheep meat industry is a product of a more recent era than, say, pig meat and grains which have deep roots in the central planning era. Thus the sheep meat industry may provide indications about how other agricultural industries can be expected to develop in the contemporary market-like environment.

The sheep meat industry has also been in the midst of China's livestock revolution, recording double digit growth rates for most of the 1990s to present. However, the sheep meat industry has grown from a low base and while China has the largest sheep – and goat – flock in the world, it still constitutes a relatively small part of the overall Chinese livestock sector. Thus the industry can be seen as a part of the diversification of China livestock production and consumption, away from traditional meats such as pig meat.

Figure 1.5 shows the growth and diversification of the meat production in China. Total meat production in China has doubled in volume every decade, so the 2004 pie graph (Figure 1.5b) is 4 times the size of the 1984 graph (Figure 1.5a). Within this high level of growth, the sheep meat industry has increased its share of production to reach 3% in 2004. When combined with goat meat (another 2%), the sheep and goat meat industries form a significant part of China's livestock sector.

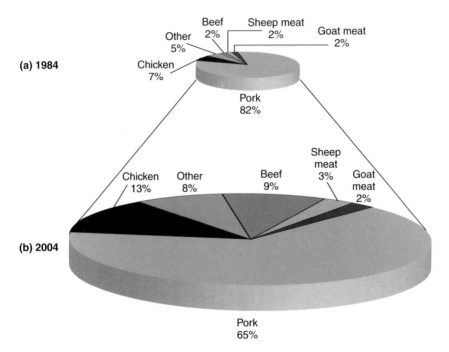

**Figure 1.5.** Breakdown of Chinese meat production by type, 1984 and 2004. *Source*: Editorial Board of the China Animal Husbandry Yearbook (various years).

The substitution between sheep meat and related commodities is another feature of the case study. Goat meat is a close and sometimes interchangeable commodity for Chinese consumers, while on the supply side wool production can be a substitute activity for both producers and traders. This poses several research problems that are applicable to other livestock industries with substitute products (such as cattle and buffaloes, and poultry meat and egg production).

Because of the recent development of the Chinese sheep meat industry, little research has been conducted on the industry. A review of the English language publications reveals scant reference to the industry. Chinese language studies on the sheep meat industry cover only limited aspects of the industry such as statistics, company profiles and developments in certain provinces.[4] The intent of this book is to provide an extensive and rigorous analysis of the industry. Apart from the insights this sheds on broader livestock industry development, the book should be a valuable reference for readers specifically interested in the Chinese sheep meat industry.

This analysis of the sheep meat industry has benefited from previous work by the authors on the Chinese wool industry (Longworth and Williamson, 1993; Longworth and Brown, 1995; Brown *et al.*, 2005), the Chinese beef industry (Longworth *et al.*, 2001; Brown *et al.*, 2002a; Waldron *et al.*, 2003), the Chinese dairy industry (Zhang, 2005), the full suite of ruminant livestock industries in China (Deng and Zhang, 2005) and in China's western grasslands (Brown *et al.*, 2007). Although differences exist between the sheep meat industry of today and these other ruminant livestock industries at an equivalent stage of development, there are also striking similarities. All of these industries underwent rapid growth in initial stages, fuelled by the potent mix of anticipation of market developments and policy-push forces. As the policy attention and speculative activity diminishes, this initial growth period is inevitably followed by a period of industry rationalization and correction. The industry then falls back on a more fundamental set of drivers based on underlying market demand, and develops at a more sustainable pace. The challenge for all these industries is to develop and access higher value market segments, especially mid value segments accessible to household producers. Although the sheep meat industry is in the early stages of development, it already displays characteristics of the cycles that have beset other ruminant livestock industries in China.

---

4. See Yao *et al.* (2002) for an analysis on the sheep (and also goat) meat industry in Gansu; Kui (2002) on Qinghai; Sun (2002) on Ningxia; Zhang and Pan (2002) and Ba *et al.* (2001) on Inner Mongolia; Yin (2002) on Jiangxi; Zhao *et al.* (2002) on Liaoning; and Chen and Chen (2002) on Xinjiang. These journal and magazine articles overview the sheep and goat industry of particular provinces in rather broad terms with little integration of (official) statistics with local level policy and agribusiness developments. However, some articles discuss the provincial sheep and goat industries around themes such as the extension system (Yao *et al.*, 2002), the market (Zhang and Pan, 2002) and trade (Zhao *et al.*, 2002).

# 2
# Statistical issues

A critical analysis of statistical indicators is important for two main reasons. First, as indicated in Chapter 1, there are concerns about the extent to which these indicators reflect the reality of industry growth and development. Second, appropriate strategies and commercial and policy decisions must be made from a well informed base. Official statistics form a key component of this information base. In relative terms, official statistics draw upon a well resourced data collation and analysis process, are widely disseminated and publicly available. This ensures that a wide range of officials, commercial interests and other industry stakeholders are drawing upon a common and accessible pool of information in making assessments and decisions. Thus industry statistics are a vital part of an efficiently functioning market and administrative system. However to realize their potential, the statistics must be relevant, accurate, timely, rigorous and reliable.

This chapter explores the statistics relevant to China's sheep meat industry. It covers the three main reported areas of statistics namely production, consumption and trade. The robustness of the statistics is discussed as a guide to how they should be interpreted. Adjustments, derivations or extensions of the official statistics designed to make them more relevant or reliable indicators are also described. The discussion also alludes to trends to emerge from the statistics to the extent allowed by the limitations of these data. This chapter focuses on some of the more widely reported and used statistics. Discussion on other statistics, especially on prices and costs of production, are left to the analysis of market drivers in Chapter 3.

## 2.1 Overview of statistics

In principle, a link exists between the key statistics of production, consumption and net trade. However, in the case of Chinese livestock statistics, the data for these items are collected through different systems and are subject to various different systematic biases. Some of the biases are illustrated in Figure 2.1 and discussed in the following sections. In general, sheep numbers, and sheep and

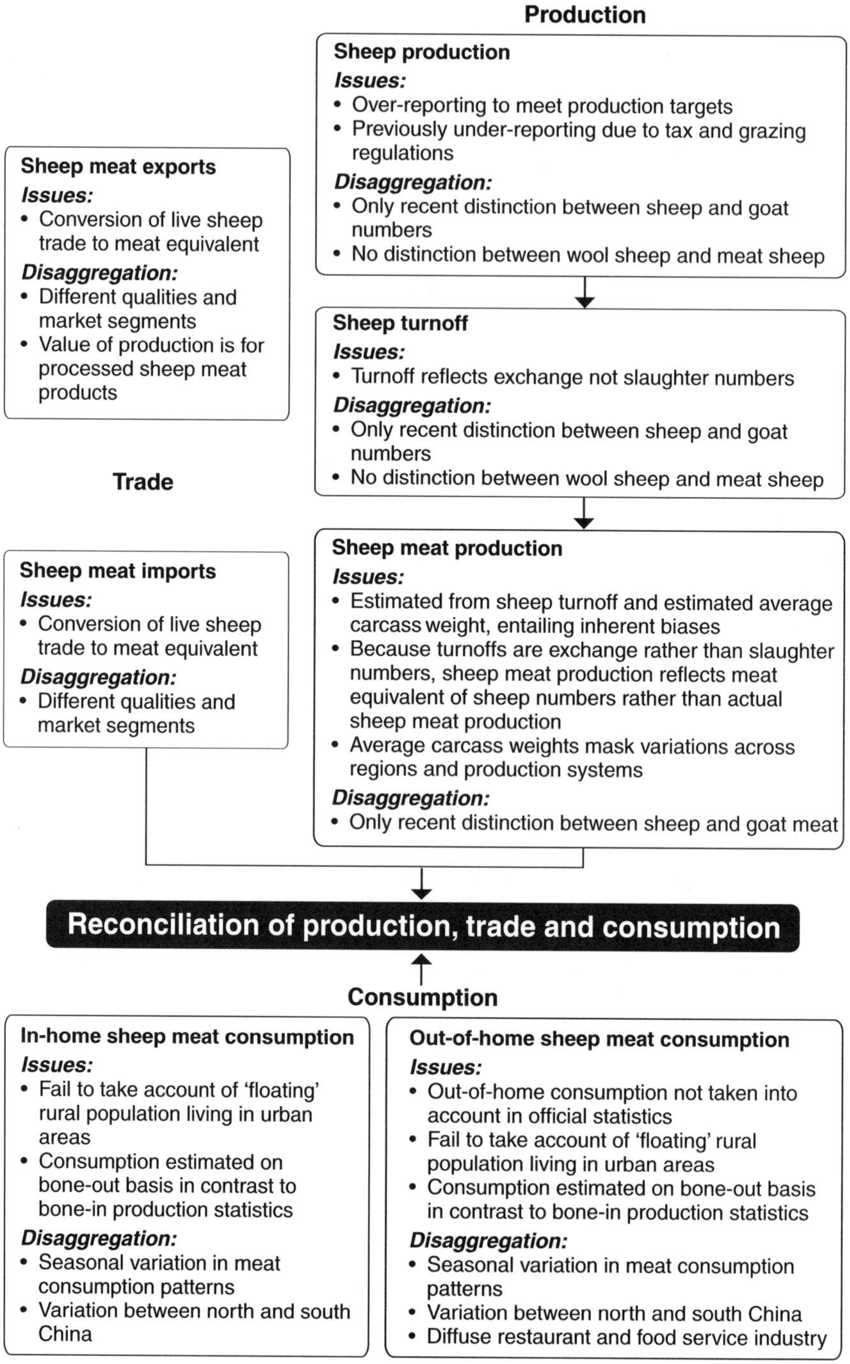

**Production**

**Sheep production**

*Issues:*
- Over-reporting to meet production targets
- Previously under-reporting due to tax and grazing regulations

*Disaggregation:*
- Only recent distinction between sheep and goat numbers
- No distinction between wool sheep and meat sheep

**Sheep meat exports**

*Issues:*
- Conversion of live sheep trade to meat equivalent

*Disaggregation:*
- Different qualities and market segments
- Value of production is for processed sheep meat products

**Sheep turnoff**

*Issues:*
- Turnoff reflects exchange not slaughter numbers

*Disaggregation:*
- Only recent distinction between sheep and goat numbers
- No distinction between wool sheep and meat sheep

**Trade**

**Sheep meat imports**

*Issues:*
- Conversion of live sheep trade to meat equivalent

*Disaggregation:*
- Different qualities and market segments

**Sheep meat production**

*Issues:*
- Estimated from sheep turnoff and estimated average carcass weight, entailing inherent biases
- Because turnoffs are exchange rather than slaughter numbers, sheep meat production reflects meat equivalent of sheep numbers rather than actual sheep meat production
- Average carcass weights mask variations across regions and production systems

*Disaggregation:*
- Only recent distinction between sheep and goat meat

**Reconciliation of production, trade and consumption**

**Consumption**

**In-home sheep meat consumption**

*Issues:*
- Fail to take account of 'floating' rural population living in urban areas
- Consumption estimated on bone-out basis in contrast to bone-in production statistics

*Disaggregation:*
- Seasonal variation in meat consumption patterns
- Variation between north and south China

**Out-of-home sheep meat consumption**

*Issues:*
- Out-of-home consumption not taken into account in official statistics
- Fail to take account of 'floating' rural population living in urban areas
- Consumption estimated on bone-out basis in contrast to bone-in production statistics

*Disaggregation:*
- Seasonal variation in meat consumption patterns
- Variation between north and south China
- Diffuse restaurant and food service industry

**Figure 2.1.** Overview of data issues in the Chinese sheep meat industry.

goat meat output are grossly overstated while sheep and goat meat consumption is understated. The difference between production and consumption can not be accounted for through net trade.

Another feature of the statistics is the common treatment of sheep meat and goat meat. Traditionally, a close substitution existed between sheep and goats on the supply side and between sheep meat and goat meat on the demand side. Indeed, the term *yang* is used to describe both sheep and goats and *yangrou* to describe both sheep meat and goat meat. Official statistics also fail to differentiate between sheep and goats in terms of scale of production, turnoff, meat production and consumption. The Ministry of Agriculture has sought to address this through special surveys and by derivation, but the unpublished results by province extend back only a single year and the two livestock species are not differentiated in widely collected or disseminated statistics.

The lack of differentiation between substitutes like sheep and goats and sheep and goat meat is a function of localized markets, low value production systems and the nature of some Chinese dishes. However, as markets become more differentiated and sophisticated, the need for a distinction becomes more pressing. Indeed the market has advanced to a stage where distinctions between lamb (sheep slaughtered at less than 1 year old) and mutton (over 1 year old) are becoming more important. Thus statistics need to evolve with market development and segmentation. Issues associated with the disaggregation of sheep and goat statistics also feature in Figure 2.1.

### 2.1.1 Source of information

Most of the data presented in this report derive from Chinese statistical yearbooks and are supplemented by other publicly available reports, magazines and internal government reports. There are essentially five sources of official statistics relevant to sheep and sheep meat: the National Bureau of Statistics (formerly known as State Statistical Bureau); the Ministry of Agriculture; the former Bureau of Internal Trade; the State Industry and Commerce Administration Bureau; and the General Administration of Customs. Within the National Bureau of Statistics, two teams – the Urban Socio-economic Survey Organization and the Rural Socio-economic Survey Organization – work on collecting, collating, adjusting and reporting the data for cities and rural areas respectively. Within the Ministry of Agriculture, a wide range of data on livestock production can be obtained from the Animal Husbandry Bureau and price information from the Ministry of Agriculture Information Centre. Import and export data for sheep and sheep meat through different ports are from the General Administration of Customs.

Three main statistical yearbooks are regarded as the official sources of statistical information on agricultural and livestock industries. The *China Statistical Yearbook* (National Bureau of Statistics, various years-b) provides an enormous amount of statistical information nationally and by province. Provincial, city and county statistical yearbooks are also available, sometimes from the National

Bureau of Statistics in Beijing, or in the capital of the region itself. These broad statistical yearbooks contain various items of direct relevance to the sheep meat industry including year end sheep numbers, annual sheep and goat meat output, and urban and rural sheep meat and goat meat consumption. The first two items are also provided in the *China Agriculture Yearbook* (Editorial Board of the China Agriculture Yearbook, various years), along with additional statistics on items such as turnoff. The *China Animal Husbandry Yearbook* (Editorial Board of the China Animal Husbandry Yearbook, various years) provides more specific live-stock related data on items such as scale of production and livestock extension stations. Both the *Agricultural Yearbook* and the *Animal Husbandry Yearbook* can be purchased through the Ministry of Agriculture in Beijing.

### 2.1.2 Official revisions to statistics

As discussed in Chapter 1, the reliability of aggregate national livestock statistics has been debated for some time both inside China and overseas. The first National Agricultural Census conducted in January 1997 collected data on the number of livestock on hand as at the end of 1996 and this allowed the traditional end of year livestock inventory estimates for that year to be checked. As a result of the census, the National Bureau of Statistics announced in late 1998 that it would revise livestock numbers and livestock output estimates for 1996 and 1997 (United States Department of Agriculture, 1998).

The national total number of sheep in stock at the end of the year for 1996 was revised downwards by 16.3% which was similar to the revision in other live-stock numbers such as bovines and pigs. However, revisions to statistics on meat output greatly exceeded those for livestock numbers, indicating that systematic statistical biases associated with livestock marketing and processing compound the biases associated with livestock numbers. Official estimates of sheep meat and goat meat output for 1996 were revised down by 27.8% as a result of the census. This was significantly more than the revisions to pig and poultry meat and slightly lower than the revision for beef output in 1996. The revisions for sheep numbers and for sheep meat and goat meat output were not uniform across provinces.

Although official revisions provide a more realistic picture of sheep numbers as well as sheep meat and goat meat output in China in 1996 and 1997, it is not clear that the systematic data collection problems have been resolved. In par-ticular, bone in sheep and goat meat output is calculated by estimating turnoff numbers and multiplying by estimated average carcass weights. For most meat output estimates to be accurate requires that turnoff numbers equate with actual slaughter numbers and that average carcass weights are genuinely representative. The accuracy of the continued sharp upward trend of livestock numbers and meat output since 1996/7 will be put to the test when the next Agricultural Census is conducted, which is planned to start at the end of 2006.

## 2.2 Production indicators

Sheep meat production (bone in) is a function of the number of sheep, the proportion of these sheep that are turned off for slaughter, and the carcass weight of the sheep slaughtered. As mentioned above, however, while sheep and goat numbers are recorded separately, official statistics do not make the distinction between the turnoff of sheep and goats and consequently between the production of sheep meat and goat meat.

Figure 2.2 presents combined sheep and goat numbers, turnoff and aggregate sheep and goat meat production for the period 1981 to 2003. Despite fluctuations, sheep and goat numbers have increased by more than 80% over the period even after a major downward revision in the 1996 census. Turnoff numbers increased at an even faster rate suggesting one or more of the following: a shift from wool sheep to meat sheep; the turnoff of younger animals; faster livestock growth rates; and higher reproductive levels. Sheep and goat meat production in turn has increased faster than turnoffs because of an increase in carcass weights or dressing percentages. The higher rates of growth in downstream industry stages are regarded in China as an important indicator of industry development and commercialization. Small changes in technical parameters, such as turnoff age or dressing percentage, can have a very large impact on aggregate outputs.

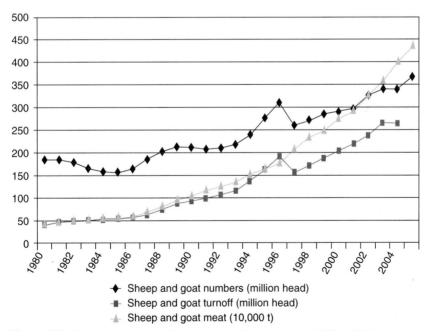

**Figure 2.2.** Sheep and goat numbers, turnoff and meat output, 1980 to 2005.
*Source*: Editorial Board of the China Agriculture Yearbook (various years). Data for 2005 is from Food and Agriculture Organization (accessed March 2006) and is provisional.

In interpreting these figures, however, it is important to be aware of some of the systematic biases in these series as they can compound the problems. Data on production aspects of the industry are collected by both the Ministry of Agriculture and the National Bureau of Statistics, both through bottom up data collection systems. Numbers of sheep in stock collected by the Ministry of Agriculture are generally overstated to over-emphasize industry development. Conversely, officials at local levels have traditionally understated statistics to the National Bureau of Statistics as these were used to determine tax and fee transfers to higher levels of government.[1]

Slaughter numbers are also overstated if assumed to equate with turnoff numbers, which is the case for statistical purposes in China. In reality, turnoff numbers represent the number of times livestock are transacted. Sheep may be sold several times through various intermediaries prior to slaughter. Thus sheep and goat meat production statistics are overstated as they are the product of turnoffs and average carcass weights. Because of the problems in interpretation, statistical yearbooks have in recent years begun to use the more specific term of 'sales and slaughter' rather than 'turnoff'.

In relative terms, sheep slaughter estimates may be more accurate than they are for cattle and beef. While sheep are sometimes traded to capitalize on trading or feeding opportunities, they are usually sold for slaughter. This compares with cattle which, particularly in agricultural areas, are often traded many times (commonly up to three times) because of their value as draught animals (Longworth *et al.*, 2001).

The estimation of average carcass weights can also create problems. Average carcass weights are estimated at local levels and fed up through the system where they are multiplied by turnoff numbers to determine bone in sheep and goat meat production. The average carcass weight for sheep in China as a whole in 2001 was estimated at 15.5 kg compared to 12.6 kg for goats. These specified average carcass weights may only broadly resemble actual average carcass weights and may not be flexible enough to keep up with changes in turnoff ages, technology or production systems.[2]

Figure 2.2 not only glosses over these statistical issues, but also the uneven spatial distribution of sheep and goats in China. At the most fundamental level, the two main sheep and goat producing regions in China are: the Western Pastoral Region (comprising Inner Mongolia, Xinjiang, Qinghai, Gansu and Tibet) characterized by extensive grazing systems; and the Central Plains (Henan, Shandong,

1. The abolishment in recent years of a range of agricultural taxes has changed reporting incentives. The abolition or reduction of various grassland taxes and fees has also meant that households in pastoral areas are more forthcoming with accurate records of their livestock numbers.
2. Carcass weights for sheep and goats combined in China as a whole increased from 13.47 kg in 2001 to 14.09 kg in 2004. Food and Agriculture Organization (last accessed March 2006) statistics estimate that average carcass weights then increased to 15.33 kg. Based on an average dressing percentage of 45%, average liveweights increased from 29.95 kg in 2001 to 31.31 kg in 2004. However, there are large inter-regional differences. For example, in 2004, the average carcass weight in Xinjiang (18.87 kg) was nearly double that of Shandong (9.61 kg).

Hebei, Shanxi, Jiangsu and Anhui), characterized by agricultural and intensive livestock production systems.

Figure 2.3 shows the distribution of sheep in 2003 and can be contrasted with the distribution in 1980 shown in Figure 2.4. Figure 2.3 reveals that sheep are distributed over a wide part of China with the exception of southern and south-eastern provinces, where there are virtually no sheep. This compares with goats which, as shown in Figure 2.5 have a much wider distribution pattern and significant numbers in southern provinces such as Yunnan, Guizhou, Hunan, Anhui and Fujian. In comparison with the distribution in 1980, sheep numbers have risen markedly in the northern parts of the Central Plains (Hebei, Henan, Shandong, Shanxi, Beijing) but have also grown markedly in the pastoral provinces of Inner Mongolia and Xinjiang and to a lesser extent in the northeastern provinces. Most of this growth has occurred only from the 1990s.

Between 1980 and 2002, the centre of sheep and goat production shifted somewhat from the Western Pastoral Region to the Central Plains agricultural areas. However, goat production has been especially pronounced in the Central Plains, which holds 46% of China's goats. Indeed some Central Plains provinces such as Anhui have moved almost entirely out of sheep and into goats. Sheep production is still concentrated in the Western Pastoral Region which is home to 64% of China's sheep.

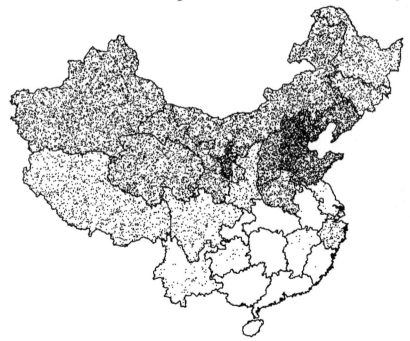

Note: 1 dot is equivalent to 10,000 sheep. The map (erroneously) assumes that sheep are distributed evenly throughout a province.

**Figure 2.3.** Distribution of sheep in China, 2003.
*Source*: Editorial Board of the China Agriculture Yearbook (2004).

Official statistics for 2003 indicate that numbers of sheep in stock in China as a whole reached 157 million head which represented an increase of 47% over the numbers in 1980. At the same time, the turnoff of 260 million sheep and goats in 2003 was more than six times that of 1980. As mentioned previously, sheep turnoffs are not distinguished from goat turnoffs in the official statistics. However, a one-off survey by the Ministry of Agriculture estimated a sheep turnoff of 81.45 million head and goat turnoff of 151.36 million in 2002, accounting for 35% and 65% respectively in total turnoff numbers of sheep and goats. The Ministry of Agriculture further advise (personal communication, 2004) that these turnoff numbers should be revised down by 5% to 6% to more accurately reflect slaughter rather than sales numbers.

Unpublished survey data of the Ministry of Agriculture in 2002 (presented in Chapter 6) also indicated that 32% of all sheep and goats were turned off by households with only one to four sheep or goats, 40% were turned off by households with between five and 49 head, 20% by households with 50 to 199 head and around 8% of sheep and goats were turned off by farms with more than 200 head. The scale of production is relatively high in the Western Pastoral Region and relatively low in southern China. Further analysis of this data appears in Chapter 6.

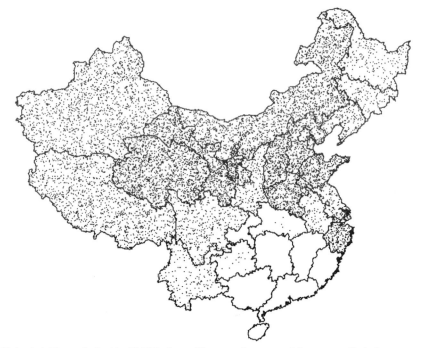

Note: 1 dot is equivalent to 10,000 sheep. The map (erroneously) assumes that sheep are distributed evenly throughout a province.

**Figure 2.4.** Distribution of sheep in China, 1980.
*Source*: Editorial Board of the China Agriculture Yearbook (1981)

The *China Animal Husbandry Yearbook* also reports scale of production data for 2003 but for different size categories. In 2003, 56% of sheep and goat turnoffs were from households turning off less than 30 sheep or goats, 28% from households with a turnoff of 31 to 100 head, 12% from households with a turnoff of 101 to 500, 3% from households with a turnoff of 501 to 1000, and only 1% from households with a greater turnoff number. The 1792 households who turned off more than 1000 sheep and goats compared with over 26.8 million households who turned off between 1 and 30 sheep and goats.

Official statistics for 2003 indicate that sheep and goat meat production reached 3,572 kilotonnes (kt), an eightfold increase on 1980 production. To estimate the output of sheep meat alone a number of factors identified in the survey mentioned above must be taken into account: there is 35:65 split between sheep and goat turnoffs; turnoff figures for both sheep and goats should also be revised down by about 5%; and average carcass weights of sheep are heavier that those of goats by about 2 kg (but can vary between 1.5 kg up to 2.9 kg as was the case in 2001). If these factors are taken into account, sheep meat output in 2003 was 1,391 kt and constituted 40.5% of the total sheep and goat meat production.[3]

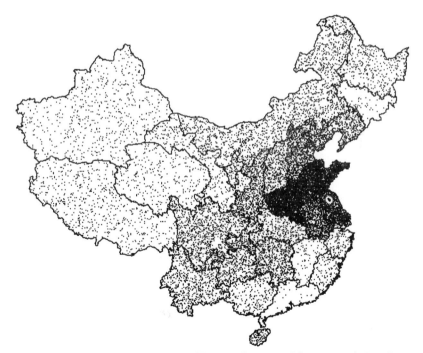

Note: 1 dot is equivalent to 10,000 goats. The map (erroneously) assumes that goats are distributed evenly throughout a province.

**Figure 2.5.** Distribution of goats in China, 2003.
*Source*: Editorial Board of the China Agriculture Yearbook (2004).

The distribution of sheep turnoffs and sheep meat production is similar to that for sheep numbers, although there are relatively fewer turnoffs compared with numbers in pastoral areas such as Qinghai and Gansu, and relatively more turnoffs in the intensive agricultural areas of Shandong, Hebei, Beijing and Tianjin.

## 2.3 Consumption

The accurate collection and portrayal of consumption statistics can be even more problematic than is the case for livestock production. Part of the problem in consumption statistics relates to the close relationship between sheep meat and goat meat in Chinese cuisine, resulting in sheep and goat meat consumption being lumped together for statistical purposes. Indeed, in some yearbooks and surveys, sheep, goat, cattle, yak and buffalo meat can be aggregated into the item red meat. This creates problems in trying to differentiate or determine actual sheep meat consumption or trends in per capita sheep meat consumption.

One way of identifying consumption is through a physical reconciliation of production and net trade – that is, where consumption equals production plus imports minus exports (on the assumption of little meat in storage). This reconciliation or supply–demand balance approach is attempted in Table 2.1 using 2002 data.[4] Sheep and goat meat production (based on carcass weights, bone in) increased from 1660 kt in 1995 to 3167 kt in 2002, or an increase of 91%. Sheep and goat meat exports increased from 1.44 kt to 5 kt over the same period, while sheep and goat meat imports increased 20-fold from 1.58 kt to 34.88 kt. Based on these figures, consumption is estimated to have increased 93% from 1656 kt to 3197 kt. This translated as an increase in per capita sheep and goat meat consumption from 1.37 kg to 2.5 kg or an increase of 82% (Table 2.1). Growth in sheep and goat meat consumption exceeds that of sheep and goat meat production over the past 7 years but virtually all consumption is still met from domestic production and not from net imports.

The National Bureau of Statistics also collects data on per capita sheep and goat meat (bone out) consumption based on surveys of between 40,000 and 50,000 households. Table 2.2 shows per capita consumption of animal products of urban and rural households in China over the period 1990 to 2002 as issued by the National Bureau of Statistics. Per capita sheep and goat meat and beef consumption of urban households decreased over the period 1998 to 2002 with per capita consumption of sheep and goat meat at its lowest level in 2002. Per capita sheep and goat meat consumption for rural areas is only half that for urban areas,

---

3. The Food and Agriculture Organization (last accessed March 2006) records sheep meat (comprised of both lamb and mutton) in China as a separate item from goat meat. The proportion of sheep meat in sheep and goat meat combined was much higher than that estimated above – 53% in 2003 and around 56% in 2004 and 2005. The accuracy of this data could not be verified.

4. A version of this method is also used in the FAOSTAT database to derive 'per capita supply'.

and consumption rates increased only slowly over the period. More recent official data from the same source indicate that per capita sheep and goat meat consumption for rural households was 0.76 kg for 2003 and 1.06 kg for 2004, while
urban households consumed 1.33 kg in 2003 and 1.39 kg in 2004. Using population weightings, this would mean a national per capita consumption of 0.9 kg in
2003 and 1.06 kg in 2004.

**Table 2.1.** Trade balance method of deriving (bone in) sheep and goat meat
consumption in China, 1995 to 2002.

| | 1995 | 1996 | 1997 | 1998 | 1999 | 2000 | 2001 | 2002 |
|---|---|---|---|---|---|---|---|---|
| | kilotonnes (carcass weight) | | | | | | | |
| (A) Production | 1660 | 1810 | 2128 | 2346 | 2513 | 2740 | 2927 | 3167 |
| (B) Export of live sheep and goats* | 4.40 | 0.94 | 0.33 | 0.24 | 0.26 | 0.24 | 0.25 | 0.12 |
| (C) Import of live sheep and goats* | 0.05 | — | — | — | — | — | — | — |
| (D) Export of sheep and goat meat | 1.44 | 1.07 | 1.31 | 2.84 | 3.46 | 4.16 | 2.87 | 5.00 |
| (E) Import of sheep and goat meat | 1.58 | 3.34 | 4.05 | 9.19 | 10.44 | 17.78 | 25.37 | 34.88 |
| (F) Net (consumption) balance (= A − B + C − D + E) | 1656 | 1811 | 2130 | 2352 | 2520 | 2753 | 2949 | 3197 |
| ***Per capita consumption (kilograms)*** | **1.37** | **1.49** | **1.73** | **1.89** | **2.01** | **2.18** | **2.32** | **2.50** |

*Calculated based on a carcass weight of 20 kg, excluding sheep and goats imported for
breeding.
'—' indicates data not available.
*Source*: Authors calculations based on data from the Editorial Board of the China
Agriculture Yearbook (various years) and National Bureau of Statistics (various years-a).

The accuracy and validity of these statistical results has been questioned by
various groups. The consumption figures are likely to be understated for at least
three major reasons. First, for both urban and rural households, only in-home
consumption is recorded thereby excluding consumption at restaurants and work
canteens and also excluding gift consumption. Second, the figures fail to account
for rural migration where between 100 and 130 million rural people are working
in urban areas. Third, the consumption of sheep and goat meat in the surveys is
calculated on a bone-out basis which is at odds with production statistics which
are calculated on a bone-in basis. Furthermore, it is intrinsically difficult for
households to give an accurate estimate of the amount of sheep meat consumed
because it forms just one of a number of ingredients in most Chinese dishes.

Despite the inaccuracies, the National Bureau of Statistics data provide
insights into regional consumption patterns. Table 2.3 shows per capita sheep and
goat meat consumption of urban and rural households by province between 1998
and 2002. Per capita sheep and goat meat consumption of urban households in
northern or western China was higher than in southern or eastern China. However,
sheep meat and goat meat consumption level increased quickly in some provinces

in southern China such as Guangdong and Guangxi. Sheep and goat meat consumption of rural households increased only moderately in provinces such as Hunan, Guangdong and Yunnan between 1998 and 2002, while sheep and goat meat consumption of rural households in northern or western China was higher than that in southern or eastern China. Overall, per capita sheep and goat meat consumption of rural households was only half of that of urban households.

**Table 2.2.** National Bureau of Statistics survey results of per capita consumption of livestock products in China, 1990 to 2002.

| Item | 1990 | 1995 | 1998 | 1999 | 2000 | 2001 | 2002 |
|---|---|---|---|---|---|---|---|
| **Urban households** | | | | | | | |
| Pork | 18.46 | 17.24 | 15.88 | 16.91 | 16.73 | 15.95 | 20.28 |
| Beef and sheep and goat meat | 3.28 | 2.44 | 3.34 | 3.09 | 3.33 | 3.17 | 3.00 |
| of which: sheep and goat meat | — | — | *1.24* | *1.23* | *1.35* | *1.25* | *1.08* |
| Poultry meat | 3.42 | 3.97 | 4.65 | 4.92 | 5.44 | 5.35 | 9.24 |
| Eggs | 7.25 | 9.74 | 10.76 | 10.92 | 11.21 | 10.41 | 10.56 |
| Fish | 7.69 | 9.20 | 9.84 | 10.34 | 9.87 | 10.33 | 13.20 |
| **Rural households** | | | | | | | |
| Pork | 10.54 | 10.58 | 11.89 | 12.70 | 13.28 | 13.35 | 13.70 |
| Beef | 0.80 | 0.36 | 0.65 | 0.54 | 0.52 | 0.55 | 0.52 |
| Sheep and goat meat | — | *0.35* | *0.63* | *0.63* | *0.61* | *0.60* | *0.65* |
| Poultry meat | 1.25 | 1.83 | 2.33 | 2.48 | 2.81 | 2.87 | 2.91 |
| Eggs | 2.41 | 3.22 | — | 4.28 | 4.77 | 4.72 | 4.66 |
| Fish | 2.13 | 3.36 | — | 3.82 | 3.92 | 4.12 | 4.36 |

'—' indicates data not available.
*Source*: National Bureau of Statistic (various years-b).

To reconcile some of the problems in estimating per capita consumption, various irregular studies have been conducted by organizations within China. One study with which one of the authors was associated was conducted by the Institute of Agricultural Economics within the Chinese Academy of Agricultural Sciences and later reported in Wang *et al.* (2004). The survey was conducted in 1998 and involved 633 urban and rural households in six provinces. In order to correct the anomalies in the National Bureau of Statistics survey design, consumption by urban households was divided into 'in home consumption' and 'out of home consumption'. Consumption by rural households was divided into 'consumption of self produced food', 'purchased consumption' and 'out of home consumption'. Sheep and goat meat as well as bovine meat are lumped together to make red meat consumption.

The survey revealed that out of home consumption accounted for 28.4% of total sheep and goat meat and beef consumption in China. Equivalent proportions were 37.5% for urban households and 16.7% for rural households. Based on these findings, the Wang *et al.* study estimated per capita sheep and goat meat consumption of all households in 1998 at 1.87 kg, with urban households having a per capita consumption of 3.5 kg and rural households 1.17 kg per capita. Based on these figures, urban residents consumed 1334 kt or 57% of all sheep and goat meat consumption in 1998, while rural residents consumed 1009 kt or 43% of all sheep and goat meat.

**Table 2.3.** National Bureau of Statistics survey results of per capita (bone out) sheep and goat meat consumption by rural and urban households by province, 1998 to 2002.

| | 1998 | | 1999 | | 2000 | | 2001 | | 2002 | |
| --- | --- | --- | --- | --- | --- | --- | --- | --- | --- | --- |
| | Urban | Rural | Urban | Rural | Urban | Rural | Urban | Rural | Urban | Rural |
| All China | 1.24 | 0.63 | 1.23 | 0.63 | 1.35 | 0.61 | 1.25 | 0.60 | 1.08 | 0.65 |
| Beijing | 4.70 | 1.10 | 4.50 | 1.00 | 4.80 | 1.10 | 4.6 | 1.20 | 4.9 | 1.30 |
| Tianjin | 4.90 | 1.30 | 4.35 | 1.30 | 4.60 | 1.10 | 4.6 | 1.00 | 4.8 | 1.10 |
| Hebei | 2.72 | 1.36 | 2.52 | 1.26 | 2.48 | 1.24 | 2.42 | 1.21 | 2.44 | 1.22 |
| Shanxi | 1.67 | 0.50 | 1.93 | 0.54 | 2.33 | 0.56 | 2.11 | 0.57 | 2.23 | 0.59 |
| Inner Mongolia | 3.46 | 2.53 | 3.31 | 2.54 | 3.60 | 2.79 | 3.31 | 2.36 | 3.38 | 2.58 |
| Liaoning | 2.35 | 0.91 | 2.05 | 0.90 | 2.01 | 1.00 | 2.06 | 0.88 | 2.00 | 0.74 |
| Jilin | 2.93 | 1.73 | 2.26 | 1.33 | 2.21 | 1.11 | 1.17 | 0.99 | 1.32 | 1.08 |
| Heilongjiang | 2.00 | 1.20 | 1.75 | 1.10 | 1.90 | 1.00 | 1.95 | 1.20 | 1.80 | 1.10 |
| Shanghai | 1.70 | 0.50 | 1.80 | 0.48 | 2.20 | 0.49 | 2.10 | 0.44 | 2.40 | 0.48 |
| Jiangsu | 0.43 | 0.47 | 0.42 | 0.32 | 0.46 | 0.23 | 0.43 | 0.21 | 0.50 | 0.21 |
| Zhejiang | 1.17 | 0.27 | 0.99 | 0.28 | 0.99 | 0.29 | 0.97 | 0.31 | 1.02 | 0.24 |
| Anhui | 0.55 | 0.24 | 0.96 | 0.22 | 0.96 | 0.21 | 0.53 | 0.23 | 0.91 | 0.26 |
| Fujian | 1.03 | 0.23 | 1.00 | 0.17 | 1.01 | 0.11 | 1.08 | 0.17 | 1.20 | 0.24 |
| Jiangxi | 1.08 | 0.22 | 0.94 | 0.18 | 1.01 | 0.12 | 1.05 | 0.17 | 1.16 | 0.23 |
| Shandong | 1.63 | 0.21 | 1.54 | 0.18 | 1.20 | 0.40 | 1.66 | 0.22 | 2.70 | 1.35 |
| Henan | 1.09 | 0.90 | 1.08 | 0.42 | 1.24 | 0.88 | 1.21 | 0.80 | 1.14 | 0.62 |
| Hubei | 0.34 | 0.40 | 0.34 | 0.39 | 0.36 | 0.27 | 0.46 | 0.33 | 0.50 | 0.35 |
| Hunan | 0.20 | 0.18 | 0.26 | 0.14 | 0.30 | 0.07 | 0.20 | 1.15 | 0.24 | 2.52 |
| Guangdong | 1.10 | 0.70 | 1.00 | 0.75 | 1.04 | 0.76 | 1.03 | 1.00 | 1.50 | 1.20 |
| Guangxi | 0.37 | 0.17 | 0.39 | 0.15 | 1.36 | 0.21 | 1.50 | 0.22 | 1.12 | 0.19 |
| Hainan | 1.02 | 0.42 | 0.98 | 0.80 | 1.10 | 0.9 | 1.03 | 0.95 | 1.04 | 0.60 |
| Chongqing | 0.33 | 0.11 | 0.30 | 0.10 | 0.36 | 0.12 | 0.42 | 0.14 | 0.45 | 0.15 |
| Sichuan | 1.00 | 0.11 | 1.02 | 0.10 | 1.13 | 0.1 | 1.02 | 0.08 | 1.20 | 0.14 |
| Guizhou | 0.75 | 0.15 | 0.55 | 0.14 | 0.75 | 0.16 | 0.65 | 0.20 | 0.74 | 0.30 |
| Yunnan | 1.30 | 0.65 | 1.30 | 0.80 | 1.20 | 1.0 | 1.20 | 0.55 | 1.30 | 1.20 |
| Tibet | 1.20 | 0.48 | 1.20 | 0.50 | 0.85 | 0.6 | 0.65 | 0.50 | 0.90 | 0.60 |
| Shanxi | 1.01 | 0.50 | 1.04 | 0.55 | 0.88 | 0.59 | 0.94 | 0.61 | 0.97 | 0.69 |
| Gansu | 1.61 | 0.52 | 1.43 | 0.25 | 1.70 | 0.02 | 1.40 | 0.01 | 1.49 | 0.38 |
| Qinghai | 7.10 | 4.60 | 6.34 | 4.70 | 7.51 | 4.5 | 7.67 | 4.40 | 6.97 | 4.60 |
| Ningxia | 5.17 | 0.55 | 4.55 | 0.53 | 6.13 | 0.33 | 4.90 | 0.45 | 5.50 | 0.50 |
| Xinjiang | 8.58 | 2.86 | 8.40 | 2.80 | 8.16 | 2.72 | 7.39 | 2.46 | 6.12 | 2.04 |

*Source*: National Bureau of Statistics (various years-b); 31 Provincial Yearbooks (various years).

For comparative purposes, Table 2.4 presents the results of the different sheep and goat meat consumption methods discussed above. Results show congruence between the 'trade balance method' and the Wang *et al.* (2004) survey results. Although not without biases of their own, results from these two estimation methods may be a better reflection of real consumption levels than those provided by the National Bureau of Statistics surveys, particularly given the glaring and significant biases in these latter surveys. If the methods and relationships from this 1998 data outlined in the Wang *et al.* study are extrapolated to 2004, sheep and goat meat consumption can be estimated to be 3.08 kg per person for China as a whole, 4.53 for urban households and 2.04 for rural areas.

**Table 2.4.** Comparison of methods for estimating per capita sheep meat and goat meat consumption, 1998.

|  | Trade balance method | National Bureau of Statistics surveys | Wang *et al.* (2004) survey |
|---|---|---|---|
| All households | 1.89 | 0.83* | 1.87* |
| Urban households | — | 1.24 | 3.49 |
| Rural households | — | 0.63 | 1.17 |

*National consumption figures derived by population weighting used by the Institute of Agricultural Economics.
'—' indicates data not calculated.
*Source*: see previous 3 tables.

## 2.4 Trade

Official trade data for sheep meat are derived from the General Administration of Customs. Items related to the trade of live animals and genetic materials also appear in the *China Agricultural Yearbook* and *China Animal Husbandry Yearbook*. Trade data on sheep meat also appear in quarterly reports issued on the Ministry of Agriculture website (www.agri.gov.cn) and in quarterly supplements in the *Peasant's Daily* newspaper.

Because of the relatively centralized import channels, China's concern with its trade balance, and in conformity with international customs conventions, relatively detailed and consistent trade data are kept.[5] More specifically, data is collected on categories of sheep and sheep products, by customs codes, as listed in Table 5.1 (Chapter 5). Data on live animal import and export distinguish between sheep and goats and between breeding stock and slaughter animals. Sheep meat is classed into various customs' categories for both fresh/chilled and also frozen product, including: lamb carcasses and half carcasses, mutton, other cuts bone in, and other cuts bone out. Goat meat is listed separately as a single category. Data for other categories combine sheep and goat offal, sheep and goat embryos and sheep and goat frozen semen, while salted sheep casings and salted goat casings are separated. For all these items, the country of origin (for imports) and destination (for exports) is listed, while various reports list the Chinese province of origin and destination.

Import and export figures for sheep meat appear in Figure 2.6. While still small in context with a domestic sheep meat production of 1108 kt, sheep meat imports rose from 1.5 kt in 1995 to 9 kt in 1998 to 30 kt by 2002. The import trade was worth US$27 million (or US$0.9 per kg) in 2002. Volumes then increased to around 34 kt in 2003, 33 kt in 2004 and 41 kt in 2005, with

---

5. Significant volumes of food, including meat, are smuggled into China mainly through Hong Kong. Despite the reduction in tariffs and dismantling of import monopolies for meat on the mainland (see Chapter 5), there are reports that this black market trade in meat continues. For more details on unofficial re-exports of beef to China through Hong Kong see Finch and Longworth (2000).

a roughly commensurate increase in value. Almost all of this imported sheep meat falls within the customs category of 'frozen bone in cuts' (not full or half carcasses), and virtually all (99%) was supplied by New Zealand and Australian exporters. In 2003, nearly all (94%) of this sheep meat was imported into the three provinces of Liaoning, Heilongjiang and Tianjin, although processors in these provinces also sell on to other areas in China.

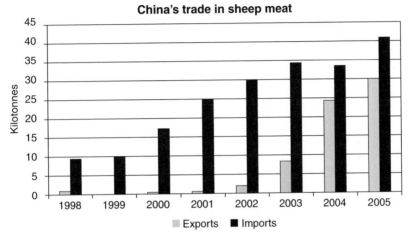

**Figure 2.6.** China's import and export of sheep meat, 1998 to 2005.
*Source*: National Bureau of Statistics (various years-a).

This trade is partially mirrored in the statistics of one of the major sheep meat exporters to China, as reported in the Australian Department of Agriculture Forestry and Fisheries Red Meat Export Statistics database (last accessed February 2006). From a negligible base, Australian sheep meat exports to China have experienced double and often triple digit growth since 1998, to reach nearly 14 kt of sheep meat (slaughter weight) in 2005. China became Australia's second largest sheep meat export destination worth AU$16 million in 2005. Virtually all of this is 'frozen bone in cuts', in particular breast flap and rack cap. This meat was imported by traders (located mainly in Dalian) and sold on to manufacturers. However, large scale manufacturers now prefer to import directly from Australian and New Zealand abattoirs, thus shortening the supply chain. The packaged product reaches the hot pot market through various channels. Final consumers can buy through retail markets or supermarkets, while hot pot restaurants can purchase direct from the manufacturer or through wholesale markets.

Australian export data suggest that the average value of sheep meat exported to China is AU$1.2 per kg (Free on Board). These prices – which convert to less than Rmb8 per kg – are about half the prices of generic sheep and goat meat in the northeast of China as reported in Chapter 3. Chinese importers incur further costs in importing, transporting, processing and packaging the product, and also generate a premium by marketing the product as imported or Australian. However, it is significant that some imported cuts are cost competitive in the Chinese hot pot sheep meat market. For the Australian industry, the trade provides a market for cuts that have little or no value in the domestic or other overseas markets (rack cap is often processed into meat and bone meal). Furthermore, separating the rack cap has increased the price of lamb racks that are sold to export markets including the United States. A similar story on a larger scale applies to New Zealand. Another feature to come from the trade data is that China imports very little goat meat.

China's increasing integration into the world sheep meat industry is also reflected in the export data. From a negligible level, China exported nearly 2 kt of sheep meat in 2002, 8.5 kt in 2003, 24 kt in 2004 and 30 kt in 2005. Until 2003 (when goat meat exports were 4 kt), goat meat exports were far larger than sheep meat exports. In 2005, exports of goat meat were about 4.5 kt, of which 3 kt went to Hong Kong. In addition to Hong Kong, the major export destinations for sheep meat and goat meat are Jordan, the United Arab Emirates and Oman. Major sheep and goat meat export provinces are Shandong, Inner Mongolia, Hebei, Beijing and Anhui.[6] Because of the low cost structures of these Chinese sheep meat abattoirs, they have been able to compete with Australian and New Zealand product in the Middle East. Exports to this price sensitive market are in carcass form, must meet Halal requirements and are destined for the retail and food service sectors.

Exports of sheep and goat offal (which are aggregated together in the data) have been negligible at less than 100 t since 1998 and fell to only 4 t in 2002 in response to high domestic demand. For the same reason, sheep and goat offal imports have increased steadily from about 500 t in 1998 to 1150 t in 2001 and 950 t in 2002, when the trade was worth US$790,000 and US$690,000 respectively. However, this trade is eclipsed by the 48 kt of beef offal imported in 2003.

Imports of sheep casing have also risen steadily from 11 kt in 1998 to 17.5 kt in 2002. The US$18 million trade was supplied mainly by Australia (10 kt) and New Zealand (4 kt) in 2002. Exports of sheep casings especially to Europe have also remained relatively constant and reached 8.7 kt in 2002, although this appears to be a lucrative trade in value terms. In recent years, China has been by far the largest market for all Australian tripe exports (up to 70%).

The trade in live sheep has also been modest in relative terms but punctuated with some significant events. China imported a total of 14,628 breeding sheep between 1997 and 2005 of which more than 80% came from Australia and nearly 20% from New Zealand. The average price of imported breeding sheep from 1997 to 2002 was US$945 per head. The data do not differentiate between

---

6. Companies in China that export sheep and/or goat meat to Middle Eastern countries include Foodstar (see profile in Chapter 7), Haoyue in Jilin (People's Daily Online, 2002a) and Jindu in Heilongjiang (People's Daily Online, 2002b).

the import of wool sheep and meat sheep, although the emphasis has certainly shifted to meat sheep for breeding purposes. Virtually no live sheep for slaughter have been imported into China.

In 1995, China exported 220,000 live sheep and goats to the Middle East. However, trade was quiet between 1995 and 2003 when China exported only small numbers of breeding and slaughter sheep and goats to Nepal, Myanmar and North Korea. Exports to the Middle East were restricted due to disease status. In 2004, live sheep exports rose to nearly 154,000 head, 93% of which went to Jordan. The vast majority of these exports are accounted for by the exports of the Caoyuan Xingfa company described in Box 7.2 in Chapter 7. In 2005, live sheep exports declined to 71,456 head, nearly all of which went to Kuwait. It is again significant that China is impinging on traditional Australian markets in the Middle East. China exported nearly 11,000 live goats in 2005, of which 7400 went to Hong Kong for slaughter in abattoirs in the autonomous region.

Apart from live breeding sheep, China has also imported significant genetic material from Australia, New Zealand and South Africa. There were 20,241 sheep and goat embryos imported between 1988 and 2003 at a value of about US$10.55 million. Embryos imported were for Dorset Down, Dorset Horn, Texel, Suffolk and Dorper sheep.

The key picture to emerge from the trade statistics is that of a small trade sector. This reflects the large size of the domestic market, the capacity of the production sector to meet this market, and the low value and localized nature of the market. From this small base, however, the trade sector is growing. Furthermore, the aggregate picture masks some of the dynamics in the industry which may alter these indicators in the future. These include the growing segmentation of the sheep meat market in China, the complementarities between the Chinese industry and other major sheep producing countries (in areas like low value cuts and by-products), the establishment of large companies with specific plans to grow exports, and the establishment of various protocols. Developments such as these are discussed further in Chapters 6 and 7 and may open opportunities for both exports from China and exports to China.

# 3

# Market forces

China's transition from a centrally planned to a market economy has been played out in the sheep and sheep meat industry. Indeed, sheep and sheep meat markets were liberalized earlier in China's market reform process than staple commodities such as grain, pigs and pork, and chickens and eggs. In this regard, the 'marketization' of the sheep meat industry is similar to the beef industry which is described in detail in Waldron *et al.* (2003, Chapter 2).

As a result of these reforms, sheep and sheep meat markets in China are relatively free and open. There are few direct administrative constraints to the trade of these commodities. Most stages of the marketing chain comprise small individual households (producers, traders, processors, retailers) which belong to the private sector and respond to market signals. Incentives that affect these households even marginally can have a dramatic impact at an industry-wide level. Thus an appreciation of market drivers is essential to understanding developments in the industry and the impacts on its participants.

The development of livestock markets in China as part of the reform process, however, does not mean that these markets operate perfectly or that there are no distortions to market signals. This is the case in the production sector where smallholders raise livestock in semi-subsistence systems, and in the trade sector where information is highly imperfect and in the extension system dominated by quasi-government agencies. Local level officials themselves are major industry players active in all industry stages. Although producers, traders and others certainly respond to market signals, they interpret and respond to signals in different ways, and assymetries of information exist between the groups.

A range of other factors also affects the way that market drivers impact on industry development. Chapters 4 and 5 reveal how market signals mix with a range of administrative signals. Even if government intervention is designed to be market conforming, markets are often poorly understood, misinterpreted and there are inevitably response lags, while market based objectives are sometimes traded off against other social and strategic objectives. As discussed in Chapters 6 and 7, the length and level of integration of marketing channels and the extent of market segmentation also influence the way by which market signals are transmitted. Technological changes can alter the relative profitability or access to production, processing and distribution activities. Thus market drivers discussed in this chapter must be seen in context with other drivers and factors discussed elsewhere in the book.

Despite the multifaceted pressures forging industry development, market drivers arguably provide the strongest indications of where the industry might be heading in the longer term. That is, institutions, policies and industry structures will change as the industry moves beyond its current, early stage of development. As the industry matures, the industry will fall back on a more fundamental set of drivers predominantly determined by market forces. These market drivers are discussed below in terms of consumer trends, prices and returns to producers.[1]

## 3.1 Consumer trends and preferences

The discussion in Chapter 2 highlighted the difficulties in determining levels of, and trends in, sheep meat consumption. Despite these difficulties, the trade balance method of estimating consumption suggested that sheep and goat meat consumption has increased significantly in recent years. Even though this method contained production-side biases, the trends identified were reinforced by data from the Wang *et al.* (2004) survey and from anecdotal evidence from knowledgeable industry participants. That is, sheep meat consumption is likely to have increased over recent years, and this acts as an important driver of industry development. Expectations that these increases will continue into the future have also encouraged industry officials and participants to invest in future production capacity.

Although such aggregate statistics and observations can be useful at a macro level, surveys of the more specific characteristics of sheep meat consumption would enable a much more detailed understanding of consumption as a driver of industry change. Detailed, relevant surveys of sheep meat consumption have yet to be conducted. However, several broader trends in food consumption in China can be applied to the sheep meat industry. Furthermore, because of the similarities between sheep meat and beef consumption, studies such as those reported in Longworth *et al.* (2001) and Cai *et al.* (1999) provide important insights into likely changes in the market profile of sheep meat.

At the broadest level, economic development and demographic change impacts heavily on food consumption patterns. A positive relationship exists between incomes and meat consumption. In China, meat consumption has increased even more rapidly than would be expected even under equivalent levels of very high economic growth in other countries. Indeed, according to Delgado *et al.* (1999)

---

1. Chinese officials and companies rarely conduct rigorous market or feasibility studies before entering into projects and plans. However, at least some reference is usually made to market trends. For an example of a study that seeks to integrate market developments with the development of the industry in Inner Mongolia see Zhang and Pan (2002).

the proportion of calories derived from livestock products doubled between 1983 and 1993, faster than for other types of food.

Surveys reported in Longworth *et al.* (2001, Chapters 13 and 14) confirm the positive relationship between increasing incomes and beef consumption in China. Similar patterns would be expected to hold for sheep meat consumption. As highlighted in Chapter 2, sheep meat consumption in urban areas is more than double that of the invariably poorer rural areas. Red meats such as sheep meat may be seen as 'superior' product although other explanations reported in Longworth *et al.* also contribute. Increased sheep meat consumption may be part of a dietary diversification away from the traditional meat diet of fat pork. Indeed, the Longworth *et al.* study establishes that the primary reason why consumers purchased beef was because it is seen as a healthy meat, and the main characteristic sought was leanness. Besides being a leaner meat than pork, sheep meat is also perceived as being produced either through extensive grazing systems (in 'green' production systems), or by small households rather than in intensive large scale feeding systems, as is more likely for pigs and poultry. Sheep have also not been associated with any widely reported disease or contamination outbreaks.

Food safety also features highly in other beef purchasing decisions of Chinese consumers. The most important quality characteristic consumers seek is freshness followed by cleanliness. Quality characteristics that are important in western countries such as tenderness and juiciness were the lowest ranked characteristics (Longworth *et al.*, 2001). These attitudes may have been forged by the nature of the product available in low value, generic markets, and the dominance of local retail markets for beef and sheep meat. This meat is sold 'wet' (rather than chilled or frozen) on the day of slaughter, but conditions at slaughter, distribution and retail can be rudimentary which cause consumers to be highly conscious of food safety issues.

Red meat is used for an enormous array of dishes and in highly varied ways (see Box 7.7 in Chapter 7). However, one of the features of sheep meat is that it forms the base of hot pot where, as discussed in Chapter 7, food is cooked in a pot of boiling water and spices on the table. Hot pot has become very popular in China in recent years because it is perceived as a convenient, social, affordable and hygienic way of eating. Because sheep meat is cooked around a pot of boiling water, and also because of traditional Chinese medicinal beliefs, sheep meat is seen as a 'hot' food, best consumed in winter and mainly in the (colder) northern parts of China. There are signs, however, that these perceptions and practices are changing.

The brief overview above suggests that consumer preferences have acted as a strong driver for growth in the industry. It also suggests that industry growth into the future will be based on a strong set of positive fundamental market forces. Furthermore, characteristics of sheep meat such as perceived health benefits and diverse forms of consumption may help in the differentiation of sheep meat within the broader food and meat industry. Ascertaining these trends requires a more detailed survey targeted specifically at consumer preferences for sheep meat.

Another broad indicator of sheep meat consumption relates to consumer expenditures. Expenditures by urban consumers on sheep and goat meat in all provinces in China between 1997 and 2001 (after which the series was terminated) were available from the National Bureau of Statistics (various years-c) and appear in Table 3.1. Expenditures generally remained steady between 1997 and 2001. This may be because of falling or stagnant prices between 1998 and 2000 or because consumption has decreased as suggested by some of the per capita consumption estimation methods presented in Chapter 2. However, the data also reveal large differences in expenditures between provinces. Annual per capita expenditures on sheep and goat meat reached Rmb193 for urban residents of Xinjiang in 2001. The next highest value of Rmb99 in Qinghai was 40% higher than the next highest region of Ningxia. Other provinces where expenditure on sheep and goat meat were relatively high were Beijing, Inner Mongolia and

**Table 3.1.** Value of urban resident per capita sheep and goat meat consumption by region, 1997 to 2001.

|  | 1997 | 1998 | 1999 | 2000 | 2001 |
|---|---|---|---|---|---|
|  |  |  | *Rmb/year* |  |  |
| Beijing | 58.41 | 55.84 | 51.77 | 54.80 | 51.03 |
| Tianjin | 46.03 | 44.22 | 47.28 | 42.52 | 40.27 |
| Hebei | 22.40 | 20.72 | 21.69 | 22.49 | 21.10 |
| Shanxi | 18.42 | 14.80 | 17.58 | 19.86 | 18.39 |
| Inner Mongolia | 43.05 | 41.45 | 40.40 | 45.70 | 46.96 |
| Liaoning | 22.61 | 21.62 | 20.31 | 25.64 | 25.32 |
| Jilin | 13.53 | 16.71 | 13.80 | 15.44 | 14.94 |
| Heilongjiang | 15.38 | 14.69 | 14.92 | 18.01 | 19.77 |
| Shanghai | 8.64 | 7.11 | 8.59 | 8.59 | 8.42 |
| Jiangsu | 6.97 | 6.06 | 6.27 | 7.66 | 6.60 |
| Zhejiang | 3.26 | 3.00 | 2.57 | 2.73 | 2.73 |
| Anhui | 7.21 | 7.71 | 9.76 | 9.55 | 7.90 |
| Fujian | 10.01 | 10.18 | 12.97 | 11.02 | 11.59 |
| Jiangxi | 0.64 | 0.67 | 0.75 | 1.04 | 0.92 |
| Shandong | 11.75 | 11.23 | 12.62 | 13.47 | 13.86 |
| Henan | 22.67 | 21.20 | 20.11 | 22.56 | 22.59 |
| Hubei | 5.55 | 4.33 | 4.11 | 5.49 | 4.49 |
| Hunan | 4.70 | 3.77 | 4.01 | 4.86 | 3.99 |
| Guangdong | 7.37 | 6.99 | 7.46 | 6.44 | 6.31 |
| Guangxi | 5.19 | 5.81 | 5.94 | 4.79 | 4.95 |
| Hainan | 12.41 | 11.20 | 15.42 | 16.57 | 14.78 |
| Chongqing | 4.28 | 2.70 | 3.42 | 4.52 | 3.87 |
| Sichuan | 3.05 | 2.46 | 3.01 | 3.36 | 3.37 |
| Guizhou | 1.67 | 1.08 | 0.86 | 1.15 | 1.34 |
| Yunnan | 2.19 | 2.04 | 1.80 | 3.38 | 3.67 |
| Tibet | — | — | 22.45 | 22.50 | 18.33 |
| Shanxi | 14.01 | 13.74 | 13.72 | 14.28 | 13.26 |
| Gansu | 19.62 | 16.83 | 15.90 | 19.44 | 17.56 |
| Qinghai | 90.56 | 86.81 | 81.47 | 90.17 | 99.39 |
| Ningxia | 75.77 | 72.32 | 64.82 | 67.82 | 69.13 |
| Xinjiang | 220.71 | 192.06 | 174.96 | 179.13 | 192.98 |
| All China | 19.25 | 17.85 | 17.58 | 18.95 | 18.97 |

*Source*: National Bureau of Statistics (various years-c).

Tianjin. These inter-regional differences confirm that sheep and goat meat consumption is much lower in southern China than northern China, especially in the Western Pastoral Region. The high expenditures in the northern and western pastoral regions of China occurred in spite of the relatively low sheep and goat meat prices (with the exception of Xinjiang).

## 3.2 Prices

Although not the only information embodied in markets, prices represent a key market signal. Price movements through time (both within and across years) have a marked impact on production revenues and consumption expenditures. Price relativities with related products in both production and consumption will also have a key impact upon decisions, as will the spatial pattern of prices which both determine and reflect the location of economic activity.

Various levels of price monitoring and price reporting occur for livestock and livestock products in China. The largest and longest series of official price data for livestock products is collected by various bodies including the Ministry of Agriculture, the Industry and Commerce Administration Bureau, and the Commodity Price Bureau. These data are collected from selected 'observation points' in markets in selected large and medium sized cities throughout China. Prices are averaged over monthly periods, to the province level and over a large number of sales to represent generic type sheep and goat meat (combined). These prices are reported in internal government reports, the *China Animal Husbandry Yearbook* in recent years, a range of television broadcasts, magazines and newspapers such as the *Peasant's Daily* on a quarterly basis. These data are presented for 1998 to 2005 in Figure 3.1 and Figure 3.2.

Although official price data provide insights into developments in the mass sheep meat market, it does not reflect developments in other market segments. The price of high value sheep meat for some cuts can be higher than that of average grade sheep and goat meat.

Figure 3.1 presents average monthly sheep and goat meat prices in China over the period January 1998 to December 2005. These monthly prices are an average of provincial prices weighted by provincial sheep and goat meat production. Because of the uneven distribution of sheep and goats in China (see Section 2.2) the weighted average provides a much more representative guide to the prices facing sheep meat producers than does a provincial average. Given that the large sheep–meat producing provinces are also large consuming areas they may also provide a useful guide to prices facing the majority of sheep meat consumers. However, the prices in Figure 3.1 may not be a good indication of sheep and goat meat prices in provinces with large consumption but little sheep and goat meat production such as some areas in south and southeast China.

The data reveal a broad price band of between Rmb13 per kg to Rmb17 per kg over the 1998 to 2003 period. Prices fell away somewhat between 1998 and 2000 but have risen steadily since then. Prices tended to exhibit more monthly variation

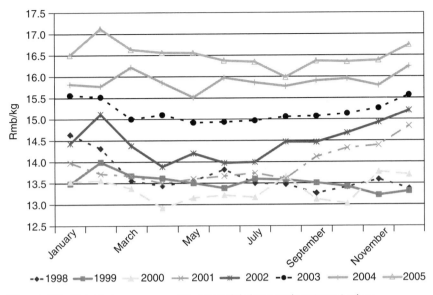

**Figure 3.1.** Weighted average monthly provincial sheep and goat meat prices, 1998 to 2005.
*Source*: Data obtained from the Ministry of Agriculture.

in the first part of the period (1998 to 2002) compared with the latter part of the period (2003 to 2005).

Traditionally Chinese people consume more sheep and goat meat in winter – especially at Spring Festival – than in other times of the year. This could be expected to lead to a seasonal pattern of prices with higher prices over the winter period from December to March, average prices in spring and autumn, and lower prices in the summer months from June to September. Although such a seasonal variation is apparent in Figure 3.1, it is relatively small with a standard deviation of monthly prices of around Rmb0.3 per kg. The variation across seasons is only slightly larger in the southern consumption regions. The relatively low seasonal variation reflects the way that the industry has developed and expanded beyond the confines of a northern and winter based industry.

Sheep and goat meat prices, however, vary more markedly across regions. Figure 3.2 reveals some of the spatial distribution of prices by reporting average prices for 2005 for all provinces except Tibet and Chongqing. Significant price variations can be observed across provinces with relatively low prices in pastoral areas of Inner Mongolia, Gansu, Qinghai, Xinjiang and Sichuan as well as in some sheep and goat intensive agricultural provinces in the Central Plains. Conversely prices are relatively high in the southern and southeastern regions where there are few sheep and relatively few goats. The variation in prices across provinces diminished slightly over the period 1998 to 2005.

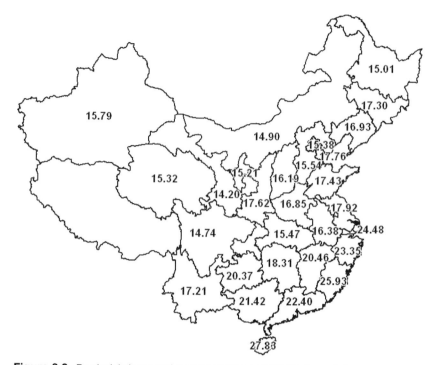

**Figure 3.2.** Provincial sheep and goat meat prices, 2005 (Rmb per kg).
*Source*: Calculated by authors based on data in Editorial Board of China Animal
Husbandry Yearbook (2004).

Brown *et al.* (2002a, Chapter 6) undertook a spatial price integration analysis
of the Chinese beef industry. The analysis investigated the behaviour of beef
industry prices in the 1995 to 1999 period, rather than the 1998 to 2003 period
investigated for sheep meat prices. However, the later development of the sheep
meat industry means that these periods are similar in terms of the stage of
industry development. The study identified some, but not complete, integration
of beef markets, as well as a broad tendency for beef price levels to converge and
become less variable as the industry developed and matured. Similar patterns are
observed for sheep meat at a similar stage of industry development.

Of more importance than sheep meat price movements, however, are the
movement of sheep meat prices relative to the prices of related commodities.
On the consumption side, a close relationship exists between sheep meat and
goat meat, while sheep meat also competes with other meats such as beef, pork
and chicken. On the production side, meat sheep compete for resources with
other livestock and farm activities. Production and substitution possibilities vary
depending on whether the sheep are being raised in agricultural areas (where
small intensively raised sheep flocks compete with other intensive livestock and

cropping activities for resources such as household labour) or in pastoral areas (where sheep compete with other ruminant livestock such as cattle and cashmere goats for scarce grassland resources). Of course one of the main substitutions and decisions made by pastoral households in particular is whether to raise sheep for meat, for fine wool, or as dual purpose sheep that produce semi-fine wool and various types of sheep meat.

Given data limitations, it has only been possible to provide price data for sheep and goat meat (combined), wool (without differentiating between types of wool) and beef. Figure 3.3 shows the price relativities between these commodities for the period since reform in 1978. The opening of markets and price reforms saw wool prices double in the 1980s. However this was much less than the rise in sheep and goat meat prices (320%) and beef (387%) during the 1980s.[3] Price relativities between wool and sheep and goat meat at the end of the 1980s and the beginning of the 1990s placed pressure on herders to switch out of fine wool and into meat sheep. Government policy aimed at promoting fine wool production slowed the rate of substitution (Longworth and Williamson, 1993; Longworth and Brown, 1995).

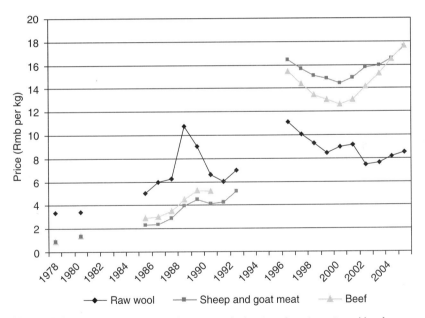

**Figure 3.3.** Mixed average prices for raw wool, sheep and goat meat, and beef, 1978 to 2005.

3. The largest increase was observed for cashmere prices which, from a low base, rose over 11-fold during the 1980s.

As these policies were either abandoned or confined to small geographical pockets, price differentials have widened even further. Although data are not available between 1993 and 1995, sheep and goat meat prices doubled annually in this period, while generic wool prices increased only moderately, meaning that by 1996 wool – sometimes known as 'soft gold' – was significantly cheaper on per unit basis than generic lumps of sheep and goat meat. All commodities entered into a decline between 1996 and 2001, but sheep and goat meat and beef recovered at a much faster rate than wool to 2005. By 2002, high international wool prices (especially for finer types of wool) had flowed on to wool prices in China but only moderately because very little of the Chinese clip is genuine Merino style fine wool.

Increasing price differentials have reinforced and intensified pressure for households – and state farms – to switch out of fine wool production and into meat sheep or dual purpose sheep production. As a result, the production of fine wool declined over the period, while the production of semi-fine wool and sheep meat increased rapidly (Brown *et al.*, 2005, Chapter 8). Furthermore, substitution back into fine wool production is a long and risky process. Indeed, large tracts of China have entered into almost irreversible breeding programmes of crossing into meat, local and dual purpose breed sheep.

## 3.3 Producer incentives

Incentives for households to raise meat sheep are an important aspect of the development of the sheep meat industry, as households raise virtually all of China's sheep. This section reports the costs and revenues associated with raising meat sheep in household production systems. Household incentives to raise sheep appear to be in line with consumption and price trends that are driving industry growth. Households in both pastoral and agricultural systems appear to have strong and growing incentives to raise meat sheep in both production systems.

Data used in this section are derived from the most widespread, comprehensive and detailed surveys of household livestock production systems in China. The data are collected by the Commodity Price Department of the new (since 2003) State Development and Reform Commission. This body was formerly called the Commodity Price Bureau under the Ministry of Planning (and several subsequent reincarnations including the State Development Planning Commission). Since the early 1980s, the Price Bureau has collected data on commodity prices and costs of production to enable price setting for a range of commodities (for the case of wool see Longworth and Brown, 1995). Although the incidence of price setting has decreased throughout the reform era, the Division continues to conduct surveys and results are published by the China Commodity Price Publishing House. One such publication is the annual *National Agricultural Products Cost and Revenues Material Collection* (Price Division of the State Development and Planning Commission, various years).

The authors collaborated with Professor Zheng Shaofeng from the College of Economics and Management within the Northwest Sci-tech University of Agriculture and Forestry to organize and analyse data related especially to livestock production systems. An overview of the analysis appears in Box 3.1. Various types of analysis based on different meat sheep production systems are discussed below. The first system investigated is an agricultural or intensive production system (Section 3.3.1) and the second is a pastoral or extensive system (Section 3.3.2). As outlined below, some overlap occurs as some of the first set of

**Box. 3.1.** Analysis of ruminant livestock production systems.

Collaborative research between the China Agricultural Economics Group at The University of Queensland and the College of Economics and Management within the Northwest Sci-tech University of Agriculture and Forestry examined data provided by the Price Department of the State Development and Reform Commission. Various types of ruminant livestock produced in different production systems were chosen, namely: i) household beef cattle in intensive agricultural systems; ii) household meat sheep and goat (lumped together) production in intensive agricultural systems; iii) specialized household local-breed sheep production in extensive pastoral systems; iv) specialized household improved breed sheep production in extensive pastoral systems; v) specialized household beef cattle in production extensive pastoral systems; vi) specialized household yak production in extensive pastoral systems; and vii) specialized household dairy cattle production in intensive agricultural systems. Provinces deemed representative to four main geographic regions in China were chosen, specifically: i) Jilin, Liaoning (Northeast); ii) Shandong, Henan, Hebei (Central Plains); iii) Yunnan, Sichuan (Southwest); and iv) Xinjiang, Gansu, Inner Mongolia, Qinghai (Northwest). In addition, national level data appear as an average of all provinces engaged in each livestock or production system type. However, national averages for livestock production in pastoral systems represent an average of the pastoral provinces only. The years 1990, 1995, 2000, 2001, 2002 were chosen for provincial level analysis for all livestock types. In addition, national or regional level data were collected for 1990, 1992, 1993, 1994, 1995, 1998, 1999, 2000, 2001 and 2002 for: i) household beef cattle in agricultural systems; ii) household meat sheep production in agricultural systems; and iii) improved sheep in pastoral systems. The data are not continuous for some livestock types, years and provinces. The number of households surveyed and the physical dispersion and coverage of households within a province vary considerably for each livestock type or system, province and year. As a guide, between 15 and 45 households were surveyed in two to nine counties in each province for each type of livestock activity. When collated to the national level, between 80 and 200 households were surveyed in 20 to 40 different counties, which incorporated the production of thousands of head of cattle and tens of thousands of sheep.

For each data subset (livestock type, year and province/national entries), two tables appear, namely a summary of revenue and costs, and a detailed breakdown of physical input and overhead costs.

The validity of the data is potentially limited by a number of factors. First, the sample size of the household surveys is relatively small and may not be representative of households in the province in question. Second, data collection and reporting may have been manipulated in line with the incentives and interests of the organizations and individuals involved. Third, the survey design may be flawed. Although the authors acknowledge these potential limitations, they are not in a position to assess the full scope of these limitations and believe the risks are outweighed by the positive aspects of the data set. The positive aspects of the survey are that: i) the surveys are the most comprehensive of their type and it has not been logistically possible to conduct comparable surveys; ii) survey reporting formats are detailed and logically presented from an economics perspective; and iii) the data provide a long time series using a consistent methodology and design. The latter feature means that discernable trends – rather than absolute values – should be accurate. With some exceptions, the findings from the analysis of the data confirmed fieldwork observations and other sources of information.

surveys also includes households engaged in semi-pastoral and pastoral livestock production. Furthermore, some households in the latter survey also use agricultural land in semi-pastoral systems. Section 3.3.3 makes some comparisons between the meat sheep production in the two types of production systems.

### 3.3.1 Meat sheep and goat production in agricultural or intensive production systems

Figure 3.4 presents key cost categories and total production value for meat sheep and goat households for the period 1990 to 2002. The results have been averaged from the survey data for different provinces. The aggregation of items in each stacked bar represents 'total production value' of raising one sheep or goat. Lower sections of the bar are disaggregated into various cost categories, and combined with net income in the top section. Compared with the early 1990s, costs have more than doubled, especially due to the increasing costs of labour, concentrate feed and lamb purchase. However, production value has increased even faster resulting in a rising net income for the households.

For sheep and goat production in intensive systems for China as a whole, the production value (excluding subsidies) of one head of sheep or goat was Rmb307

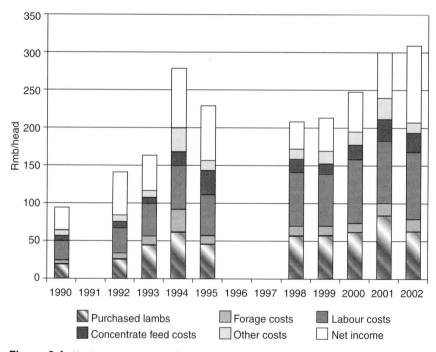

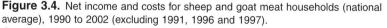

**Figure 3.4.** Net income and costs for sheep and goat meat households (national average), 1990 to 2002 (excluding 1991, 1996 and 1997).
*Source*: Authors' calculations based on data in Price Division of the State Development and Planning Commission (various years).

in 2002, while total costs (including taxes) were Rmb212, generating a net income of Rmb95. This contrasts with per head net incomes of less than Rmb40 in 1998. Increasing net income from sheep and goat production is evident in most surveyed provinces, with some exceptions in semi-agricultural systems in remote parts of China such as Xinjiang.

Net income figures for this national average as well as selected values from other provinces for various years appear in Figure 3.5. They reveal the fluctuation in net incomes throughout the 1990s and 2000s. However, there has been an increase in net incomes, especially in agricultural provinces, since the late 1990s reflecting the rise in sheep meat prices discussed in Section 3.2 above. The rise in net incomes provides households with increased incentives to enter into or expand meat sheep or goat production.

The extent of household incentives can be further explored by examining the relative profitability of alternative livestock production activities. Beef cattle production in household agricultural systems is compared with household meat sheep and meat goat production on the basis of net income per 50 kg of live weight produced in order to make the comparison possible. Figure 3.6 illustrates the relationship at the 'national average' level. The difference in profitability of cattle versus meat sheep and meat goat production appears small and varies on a year by year basis. At a provincial level, beef cattle production appears to be more profitable than meat sheep and meat goat production for provinces such as Shandong and Jilin, but the gap has diminished in recent years.

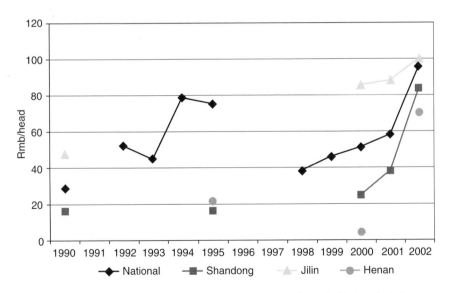

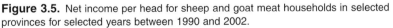

**Figure 3.5.** Net income per head for sheep and goat meat households in selected provinces for selected years between 1990 and 2002.
*Source*: Authors' calculations based on data in Price Division of the State Development and Planning Commission (various years).

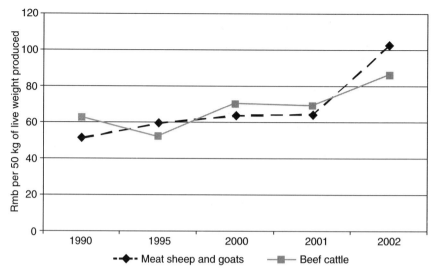

**Figure 3.6.** Net incomes (per 50 kg of liveweight produced) for beef cattle households compared with meat sheep and goat households.
*Source*: Authors' calculations based on data in Price Division of the State Development and Planning Commission (various years).

### 3.3.2 Sheep production in pastoral or extensive production systems

The survey data also incorporate the household production of two types of sheep in pastoral production systems. The first and largest category of sheep is 'local breed sheep' that produce coarse wool for local markets and where the production value is generated from natural increase and live weight gain (which together constitute total herd live weight increase). In the second category of 'improved sheep', wool production (typically semi-fine wool) accounts for a greater proportion – but still not the majority – of total production value. Limiting the survey to these two categories overlooks the category of 'fine wool sheep', many of which shifted back into the category 'improved sheep' in the 1990s (Brown *et al.*, 2005, Chapter 8). Furthermore, as mentioned in Chapter 6, many sheep breeding programmes emphasize crossing into specialized meat sheep breeds, many of which are not 'local' breeds. Nonetheless the two categories of local sheep and improved sheep currently dominate household production systems in the pastoral region and so provide useful insights into the incentives and some of the choices facing most producers.

The analysis of local breed sheep used for meat production for provinces in the pastoral region reveals that production value (from natural increase, live-weight gain and sheep value) steadily increased, while some costs (especially labour, forage and concentrate feed) have decreased in recent years. In 2002, total production value was Rmb130 per head, total costs were Rmb53, leaving a net income of Rmb77 per head. This contrasts with a net income of Rmb25 in 1995. These average results suggest that the profitability of raising local breed sheep is increasing for households in pastoral areas.

Figure 3.7 compares net income (per 100 head of sheep) for the local breed households with that for households with improved sheep. The figures are for an average of the surveyed households and provinces in the pastoral region. They reveal that the net income of the improved sheep households was larger for most of the 1990s although the gap narrowed or disappeared in the early 2000s. Further disaggregation of the costs and revenues reveals that revenues from the natural increase and live weight gain of local breed and improved sheep households are similar. Thus the higher net incomes for the improved sheep households reflect the fact that the semi-fine wool revenues generated exceeded the additional costs of raising these improved sheep relative to the local breed sheep.

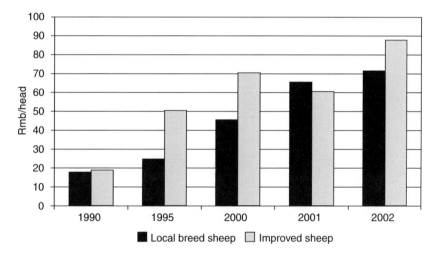

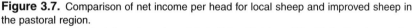

**Figure 3.7.** Comparison of net income per head for local sheep and improved sheep in the pastoral region.
*Source*: Authors' calculations based on data in Price Division of the State Development and Planning Commission (various years).

### 3.3.3 Comparison of meat sheep and goat production in agricultural areas and local breed sheep in pastoral areas

A final form of analysis that may provide some insights into the likely geographical growth for meat sheep production is to make a two-way comparison between net incomes for meat sheep and meat goat production in agricultural areas, and local breed sheep production in pastoral areas. Different accounting and survey items make the comparison problematic. Nevertheless, Figure 3.8 makes a simple comparison using averaged data for areas that fall into the two systems.

One aspect to emerge from Figure 3.8 is that net incomes for sheep and goat meat producers in agricultural areas exceed that of local breed sheep producers in pastoral areas in most years since 1990. This may help explain the remarkable increase in sheep and goat production in agricultural areas which has risen faster than sheep production in pastoral areas. However, comparative advantage may be more important than absolute advantage in driving regional developments in the industry. That is, although net incomes from meat sheep production may be higher in absolute terms in agricultural areas, they may be lower in comparative terms to the net incomes from other (on- and off-farm) activities in agricultural areas. Thus many households in the pastoral region have substituted out of other livestock products and into meat sheep production, which has driven the substantial growth in the industry in pastoral areas.

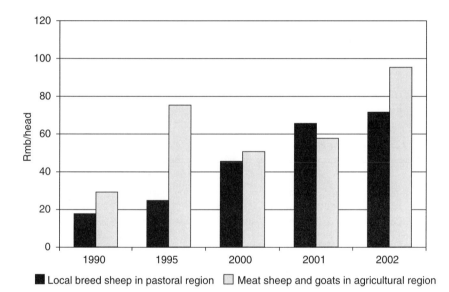

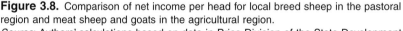

**Figure 3.8.** Comparison of net income per head for local breed sheep in the pastoral region and meat sheep and goats in the agricultural region.
*Source*: Authors' calculations based on data in Price Division of the State Development and Planning Commission (various years).

# 4

# Institutional changes

Institutional settings described in this chapter underpin policies examined in the next chapter and the agribusiness and industry developments analysed thereafter. As such, institutions can be regarded as industry drivers. This is especially the case in Chinese agriculture where some powerful institutions have a strong capacity to directly and proactively influence industry development. In contrast, other institutions – involved in activities such as market facilitation and environmental regulation – are more notable for their lack of capacity, which also affects the way agricultural industries develop.

Navigating the vast network of institutions relevant to industry development is important but problematic. The number of institutions and the rate of change make it difficult to clarify their roles and relationships. It is even more difficult to identify their effect on industries. In light of these problems, various frameworks can be drawn upon to examine the role of institutions. Waldron *et al.* (2003, Part B) detail the institutional hierarchy for the Chinese beef industry on the basis of their horizontal and vertical (*tiaotiao kuaikuai*) relationships. Waldron *et al.* (2006) overview the change in state – administrative, service, and enterprise – structures for the agricultural sector as a whole. Brown *et al.* (2005, Chapter 3) overview institutional change with a special emphasis on testing and standards institutions in the wool industry.

This chapter uses a condensed and hybrid approach comprised of horizontal structures, vertical structures, local group structures and the enterprise sector. The analysis shows that state institutions in agriculture have a strong capacity and mandate to proactively guide the development of industries and sectors as well as to absorb or coerce other non or quasi state actors to participate in the process.

## 4.1 Horizontal structures

In the central planning era and well into the 1990s, a large number of so called 'specialized economic departments' exercised economic functions in the industries with which they were associated. Rather than having jurisdiction over industries as a whole, jurisdiction was distributed along sectoral lines. The agricultural inputs sector was controlled by the Ministry of Agriculture and the Ministry of Internal Trade, the production sector was governed by the Ministry of Agriculture, processing was the responsibility of the Ministry of Internal Trade and the Ministry of Light Industry, marketing was controlled by the Ministry of Internal Trade, and trade was administered by the Ministry of Trade and Economic Cooperation with some additional roles for the Ministry of Agriculture.[1]

Because of both the overlaps and artificial distinctions in the system, government reform measures abolished or downgraded all of the above government bodies with the exception of the Ministry of Agriculture. As one of the only specialized economic departments to have survived the reforms, the Ministry of Agriculture has a mandate to proactively guide the development of the agricultural sector. This mandate is particularly strong in its traditional 'turf' in the production, inputs and extension aspects of agriculture. However, the abolition of competing specialized economic departments has allowed the Ministry of Agriculture to move into new areas such as processing, marketing and the integration and development of entire agricultural industries. Thus more than other periods in China's modern economic history, a single government department – the Ministry of Agriculture – has wide-ranging jurisdiction over most aspects of most agricultural industries.

### 4.1.1 The Ministry of Agriculture and Animal Husbandry Bureau

The Ministry of Agriculture is an enormous and diverse bureaucratic organization, comprised of 19 subordinate administrative bodies that design and implement the policies discussed in Chapter 5.[2] Poverty alleviation programmes are administered by the State Council Poverty Alleviation Office housed within the Ministry of Agriculture. The Food Safety and Quality Centre administer a series of other certification schemes, including the 'Green Foods' system and the 'Safety Foods' system. The Policy and Law Department is responsible for drafting laws crucial to the agricultural sector such as the grassland, cooperative, feed and livestock laws. Various bodies including the Vertical Integration Office administer the vertical integration programme.

---

1. The titles of these institutions changed in various periods, and there were a range of subordinate bodies and agencies that implemented state work in their designated areas of the economy.
2. Bodies under the Ministry of Agriculture include: Policy and Law Department; Market and Economic Information Department; Rural Economy System and Management Department; Development Planning Department (including the Agricultural Resource Regional Planning Office); Cropping Management Office; Land Reclamation/State Farm Bureau; Aquaculture Bureau; and the Animal Husbandry Department (including the National Feed Work Office). The Veterinary Bureau was split from the Animal Husbandry Bureau as an independent entity in 2004. The Office of the State Council Leading Group on Poverty Alleviation Development is housed within the Ministry of Agriculture. Each of these bodies also has its own subordinate structure. Far larger hierarchies exist at local levels and can vary from central level structures. There are another 46 service units (*shiye units*) and 54 professional organizations (*yewu shetuan*) under the Ministry of Agriculture at the central level.

Although these bodies are important in setting the environment in which agricultural activity takes place, the department most directly influencing livestock and the sheep meat industry is the Animal Husbandry Department. Formerly known as the Animal Husbandry Bureau at the central level, it is still known by this title at local levels. Within the Animal Husbandry Department/Bureaus, the Animal Husbandry Division and the Industry Development Division develop industry plans, targets and programmes. The Grasslands Division develops grassland policies relevant to livestock production in pastoral areas, while the Feed Division (including subordinate bodies such as the Straw for Ruminants Office) develops feed policies and programmes.

At the central level Animal Husbandry Department there are few officials with expertise in sheep and goats. However, in sheep intensive regions with a history in the industry, there can be several sheep experts in, say, a county level Animal Husbandry Bureau. These cadres usually have a technical background (as animal scientists or veterinarians) and play a key role in developing policy toward the industry and advising higher level, more general, policy makers. This partly explains the tendency for government to emphasize production rather than management or economic aspects of the industry.

While the Animal Husbandry Bureau is involved in a wide range of activities, it focuses primarily on livestock production. The most important body is the Animal Husbandry (Production) Division which, as an administrative unit, makes industry plans and policies. The separate task of delivering livestock production services – such as breeding, feeding and veterinary services – is the responsibility of a service hierarchy called the Animal Husbandry and Veterinary Centre, along with its local level stations which come under the control of local government.[3]

As is the case with all state structures, there is a distinction between administrative units and service units. In theory the two units are linked through 'professional relations' rather than the stronger 'leadership relations' that link higher and subordinate units. In practice, however, administrative structures have a major influence on the activities of service units such as those in the extension system, associations, and monitoring, testing, standards, information and research centres.

### 4.1.2 Other departments

Another major element of China's government reform programme has been to create and elevate a series of 'macro control departments' that play a broader and more 'passive' role in the economy than do specialized economic departments. The Ministry of Agriculture and the Animal Husbandry Bureau have been forced to share some of their responsibilities with the new macro control departments.

---

3. For an overview of institutional aspects of the China livestock health system see Bedard and Hunt (2004).

For more strategic tasks such as planning and agricultural adjustment, the Ministry of Agriculture must work alongside the State Council itself, the Economic and Trade Commission at local levels, the National Development and Reform Commission and the (new) Ministry of Commerce. For more specific tasks, related bodies include the Industry and Commerce Administration Bureau (for the administration of companies, traders and markets), the Administration for Quality Supervision Inspection and Quarantine (for international and some inter-regional inspection), the Ministry of Health (for food and vendor inspection), the Environmental Protection Bureau (rural environment and resource management including grasslands), the National Bureau of Statistics (including statistics in agriculture) and the Ministry of Science and Technology (for technical extension).

The creation and elevation of these macro control departments suggests that China is creating a set of institutions that are less interventionist in nature and more like those seen in developed market economies. The continuation of the development of market related institutions is critical in the development of markets and regulation of Chinese agricultural and livestock industries. However, this is occurring from a low base and is a long term undertaking. The macro control departments are not as focused on the activities of particular industries as are specialized economic departments and so do not influence the industries as strongly. Furthermore, given the priority afforded to rural and agricultural development and modernization in China, high level Party and state leaders are unlikely to relinquish interventionist controls such as those held by the Ministry of Agriculture.

## 4.2 Vertical structures

High level institutional settings discussed above are merely 'shells' – just as central level policies discussed in Chapter 5 are merely rhetorical 'mirages' – if they are ineffectual at local levels where the vast majority of agricultural activity takes place. Thus it is important to examine the strength and nature of these vertical structures and relationships. Vertical structures in Chinese livestock industries are strong only if matched with the necessary discipline and resources. This is often but not always the case in Chinese agricultural industries including sheep meat.

The Ministry of Agriculture and the Animal Husbandry Bureau administrative hierarchy is one of the few in China to be required by the State Council to extend from central down to township levels (Burns, 2003). Beyond the formal hierarchies of these administrative systems, a range of further institutions at village level and below exist that are incorporated within the broader agricultural system. These include village officials (who are usually Party members with an affiliation with the agricultural system and township government), the official extension system (part of the Animal Husbandry and Veterinary Service system that extends to village level), local group activities (including 'small areas' and associations) and enterprises.

Although the Ministry of Agriculture is large and diverse, it also forms a monolithic hierarchy. The official appointment system provides disciplinary levers (the 'stick') for higher levels of government to generate desired outcomes at local levels of government. The system also allows for the disbursement of favours ('carrots') to a range of industry actors to encourage compliance. These carrots are particularly attractive in poor, 'investment hungry' parts of China which is where the sheep meat industry has grown most rapidly in recent years.

This diverse range of actors that makes up the agricultural system has been motivated not only by the market drivers discussed in Chapter 3, but also by the policy drivers discussed in Chapter 5. With regard to the latter, policy makers wield a set of carrot and stick instruments to generate desired policy outcomes at local levels.

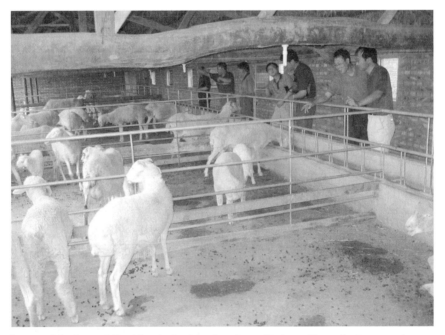

**Image 4.1.** A specialized livestock raising 'small area' in Inner Mongolia. A group of county level Animal Husbandry Bureau officials inspect the pens that the Bureau helped build for a Small Tailed Han sheep small area in Chifeng Prefecture.

However, it can also be argued that the strength of both the carrot and stick incentives in the vertical hierarchy is diminishing in China. The strength of the stick has been diminished by: fiscal reforms that have increased localized power vis-à-vis the Centre; administrative reforms that have diminished the interventionist powers of government departments; commercialization of the extension system (where state extension units are less reliant on government for funding, and non state actors have entered into areas such as breeding on a commercial basis); enterprise reform measures (that have reduced the reliance of enterprises on the state); and the freer association of local farmer and marketing groups. With rural and regional development, the carrot instruments also have had to become more generous to provide incentives for participants to comply. Thus policies and decrees not matched with the necessary resources are unlikely to mobilize industry actors on a large scale or scope.

Because of the complex and changing nature of vertical relationships in Chinese agriculture, it is difficult to interpret the efficacy of many policy edicts and statements made at a high level. These messages need to be interpreted on a case by case basis, as is done in Chapter 5.

## 4.3 Industry organizations and local groups

In addition to the government organizations overviewed above, non or quasi government organizations also play an important role in industry development, especially industry integration and coordination. Two major forms are overviewed here, namely industry associations and local groups. Although the numbers of such groups have proliferated in China in recent years, they are not as strong or independent as their counterparts in developed market economies.

### 4.3.1 Industry associations

Most industry associations in China see their roles as providing a link between government and enterprises. Indeed, many large industry associations have a background as government departments. For example, the China Meat Association, formerly under the Ministry of Commerce/Ministry of Internal Trade, helped coordinate the large number of state owned abattoirs known as General Food Companies. With the abolition of the ministry, and the divestment and corporatization of the state owned abattoirs, the association has become a more independent body that falls within the new Ministry of Commerce and registered under the Ministry of Civil Affairs. It is reliant on the same group of about 500 enterprises for most of its fees in return for the provision of industry services such as information, exhibitions and representation. The association struggles to survive and make worthwhile contributions to the industry without sufficient resourcing from, for example, levies on members which are not mandatory in China.

Livestock associations exist from central down to very local levels. They are registered with the Ministry of Civil Affairs but are still closely linked to administrative units in the Agriculture and Animal Husbandry hierarchies and are often staffed by former Animal Husbandry Bureau officials. One large association at the central level called the China Animal Agriculture Association, which was established in 2001, has a sub-association for sheep and goats. In some provinces such as Shandong, the provincial livestock association is divided into provincial sub-associations that focus on particular livestock types, including sheep and goat meat. Some of these government-orchestrated associations have branches down to city levels, such as the Heze Sheep and Goat Association, or to county level as in the case of the Liangshan Small Tailed Han Sheep Association.

Another example of an industry association is the China Sheep Association. This is a service unit under the Inner Mongolia Department of Science and Technology. Like most service units, it has a mandate to earn extra revenue on a fee for service basis. It has about 200 members (including feedlots, breeders and processors) that pay membership fees for services such as research, training, publications, exhibitions, marketing services and access to a website.[4]

Another notable development is that companies have also taken a role in developing industry associations. For example, the Dongying Beef Association in Shandong is organized by the Hengdian Company, which has an abattoir based in Zhejiang Province. The Daxing Mutton Sheep Association revolved around the Kangda Group on the outskirts of Beijing.[5] In these cases, local associations become the means of organizing livestock inputs and coordinating with households as well as other industry stakeholders.

### 4.3.2 Local groups

At another level down, the number of small local (village and township) groups in China comprised mainly of households, has proliferated rapidly in recent years (Shen *et al.*, 2004). Local group structures aim to coordinate the activities of a large numbers of households so that they can supply the quality, homogeneity and quantity of commodities required by downstream actors, especially abattoirs that target higher value markets. Many forms of local level groups exist, including informal specialized villages, farmer associations, 'small areas' and informal cooperatives. These local group structures have incorporated large numbers of farmers including those involved in sheep production. In part this is related to a policy of specialization overviewed in more detail in Chapter 5. Local groups can be influenced to serve the interests of local government and enterprises.

## 4.4 Enterprises

A final form of institutional structure relates to enterprises of which there are many types in the sheep meat industry. Notionally, enterprises in the sheep meat industry have undergone reform and liberalization in line with broader enterprise reforms. Regardless of ownership type or size, however, enterprises encountered in the sheep meat industry invariably have close relationships with government

---

4. See www.chinasheep.com.
5. The company used to maintain a website and information centre called the China Sheep Network on www.sinosheep.com but, as with the company and association, this network was disbanded in 2005.

at the corresponding administrative levels as a result of the forces explained below. More detail on specific enterprises and their activities are provided in Chapters 6 and 7.

### 4.4.1 General Food Company abattoirs

The sheep meat industry has historically comprised several types of state-owned enterprises. The several hundred relatively large and mechanized or semi-mechanized sheep abattoirs under the General Food Company system were particularly significant in the industry. The legacy of this system continues today in the slaughter, storage and transport sectors. The General Food Company abattoirs (*roulianchang*) were set up to service Muslim minorities, to promote exports (mainly to the former Soviet Union) and in response to fiscal reforms in the 1980s that encouraged local value adding. With over-capacity in the sector, enterprise reforms and the abolition of the parent government department – the Ministry of Commerce/Ministry of Internal Trade – companies were forced to become increasingly autonomous. The vast majority of these abattoirs have been closed, leased out, sold outright, or sold partially in which case local government retains part of the remaining abattoir. Many General Food Company abattoirs that slaughter sheep were sold or leased to the Caoyuan Xingfa Company as overviewed in Box 7.2, while abattoirs in the beef sector are discussed in detail in Waldron *et al.* (2003, Chapter 7).

### 4.4.2 State farms and breeding stations

There are various types of state farms but the two most important were those belonging to the Ministry of Agriculture (under the State Land Reclamation Bureau) and the Production and Construction Corps (see Longworth *et al.*, 1993). State farms have traditionally been significant actors in the sheep industry – fine wool in particular – because of their well developed breeding programmes and scales of production. This level of importance has changed with the reform of state farms. State farm management has more freedom to decide the activities they pursue rather than being forced to follow administrative decrees. In many cases, this has meant a move out of breeding activities, although some retain substantial 'core' breeding sheep flocks for commercial reasons. Furthermore, households on the state farms have increased independence – through land contacts and livestock ownership – to decide their own economic activities. In many cases, this facilitated a move out of purebred sheep meat production toward mixed flocks. Either way, state farms are no longer a primary vehicle for implementing breeding policies for ruminant livestock industries. Statistics on the number of sheep on state farms appear in Chapter 6.

Sheep breeding stations are service units of the Animal Husbandry Bureau system but are under the direct leadership and are funded by local government. As discussed in more detail in Chapter 6, there are approximately 450 breeding stations for meat sheep types in China. They are subject to similar reform measures as those of state farms and are eligible to become fully fledged companies as a means of easing financial demands on local government. In many cases, these stations have been bought out by the former staff and then run as a commercial breeding venture. Similar examples arise in the case of veterinary stations and other forms of livestock service stations.

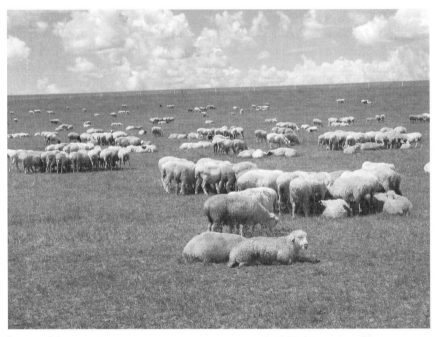

**Image 4.2.** Sheep flock on state farm in Inner Mongolia. While most sheep on state farms have been distributed to households which have been shifting out of fine-wool sheep production, state farms retain core fine-wool sheep breeding flocks such as those pictured. In many cases, however, these core breeding flocks are also being oriented toward meat sheep breeds.

### 4.4.3 Other enterprises

The reform of state structures and entrepreneurialism by former staff of state-owned enterprises has been supplemented by the entry of new actors into the sheep meat enterprise sector. The vast majority of these actors are small individual households or groups of households that have formed production, marketing, slaughter or processing companies. The development of the sheep meat industry, however, has also encouraged the entry of enterprises that are significant on national and provincial scales, and have structures that range from collective to shareholder to private companies.

Government bodies keen to create development opportunities actively encourage the development of 'scale' enterprises regardless of their ownership structures.

This is particularly the case for enterprises active in what are regarded as emerging industries such as sheep meat. Such enterprises are offered numerous forms of assistance from government at different levels. Preferential policies for a large central level sheep meat enterprise included a waiver of profit taxes. For more local level enterprises, resources such as land are provided by local government. Enterprises are very often incorporated into local development projects targeting poverty alleviation or specialization.

The most important and tangible forms of assistance provided by government, however, is in the form of services and organization. For example, abattoirs receive assistance to source required sheep from large numbers or groups of households which are organized, trained, and provided with extension services and infrastructure by government. Breeding companies very often sell breeding sheep to households with credit organized by local government for poverty alleviation projects. Further details on government–business relations are provided in the discussion of policies in the next chapter, while the failure of many large enterprises in the industry is discussed in Chapters 6 and 7.

# 5
# Policy initiatives

Institutions described in the previous chapter employ a range of policy instruments to achieve various social and strategic objectives. These policies can be pursued to correct market failures, to pre-empt future market forces, to facilitate the environment in which the market operates or to overcome the perceived adverse outcomes of the market drivers discussed in Chapter 3. Thus policy drivers, and their interaction with market and institutional drivers, can not be overlooked as a force in forging industry development.

Navigating the enormous number of policies relevant to agricultural industries in China can be a daunting task. Policy edicts and announcements give the impression that the policies are large, well resourced, coordinated and have a high impact. Although this can be the case, many other policies are undertaken on a trial basis, are rhetorical in nature – a 'policy mirage'[1] – or are implemented unevenly. This chapter seeks to categorize policies relevant to the sheep meat industry and to analyse them in a critical manner.

Four categories of policies are examined: sectoral and industry policies; social and environmental policies; market support services; and trade policies. Within this suite of policy instruments, most emphasis in China is given to the first category of sectoral and industry policies that are 'top down' and interventionist in nature. They are intended to fuel the initial rapid growth of the industry and to meet various strategic and social objectives. They are afforded more attention than are market support services which will need increased emphasis to facilitate the longer term development of the sheep meat industry.

## 5.1 Sectoral and industry policies

China wields a range of top down or interventionist policies to guide economic and rural development. Many of these policies are directed at the agricultural

---

1. Longworth and Williamson (1993) used the term 'policy mirage' to refer to situations where local-level decision makers were unaware of, overlooked, or implemented differently policy edicts from higher levels.

and livestock sectors and are intertwined with policies targeted at particular industries including sheep meat. Considered together, this suite of policies change incentives for industry actors, including households, companies and local government. This is particularly so in the early stages of industry development as is the case for the sheep meat industry. Policies fast track industry development not only in terms of production and output, but also toward increasing scale, quality and modernization.

### 5.1.1 Industry plans and adjustment policies

Under China's economic reform programme, rigid central planning has given way to plans or targets that 'guide' growth and development. Most apparent are the formal 5 year plans but they are also made on a shorter term basis including annual plans. Plans are drawn up from the central down to the village level. Officials lower down the hierarchy are under pressure to fulfil higher level targets, and thereby increase their chances of promotion. However, local officials also develop their own set of more specific and often more ambitious targets.

Officials from various government bodies such as the Economic and Trade Commission, the Ministry of Agriculture and the Animal Husbandry Bureau draw up livestock industry plans. Specific industry plans (such as for sheep meat and goat meat) are incorporated into sectoral plans (livestock and agriculture) and into the broader economic plan for the region. However, because institutional structures are often disjointed and not well integrated in China, and because individual institutions hold strong and independent decision-making powers, policies are often made in isolation with little consideration for what is happening in other regions or sectors of the economy. Some examples of government output plans or targets involving sheep are highlighted in Box 5.1.

Most plans focus on increasing output, especially sheep numbers, turnoff and sheep meat production. Part of this is a legacy of the central planning and early reform eras where agricultural commodities were generally under-supplied. Now that surpluses have set in for virtually all agricultural commodities at national and regional levels, emphasis is beginning to change toward improving commodity quality, industry modernization and international competitiveness, including in the processing sector. In Chinese terms, this involves 'optimizing and restructuring' agricultural industries and 'upgrading' China's agriculture.

A catch-all programme that incorporates these objectives is known as 'strategic adjustment of agricultural structures' (*nongye jiegou zhanluexing tiaozheng*). This programme has impacted on both the cropping and livestock sectors and on the relationships between the two sectors. It has been applied to upstream segments (pre-production and feed) and downstream segments (processing, marketing and distribution). In the cropping sector, emphasis has turned toward higher value crops (such as high value soybeans and cotton) mainly because these commodities have been imported in significant quantities in recent years and import replacement and national self sufficiency remains an important national priority.

**Box 5.1.** Examples of local industry plans in the sheep meat industry.

Chifeng City, a populous semi-pastoral prefecture-level city in eastern Inner Mongolia, had 6.7 million sheep and goats in stock at the start of 2004 with a turnoff of 3.3 million head. The industry was 'grabbed' for development in 2003 and ambitious targets set. The prefecture aimed to have 10 million sheep and goats by the end of 2004 and 30 million by 2008 with a turnoff of 12 million head in the same year. By the end of 2005, however, the prefecture had fallen well short of the plans. Indeed numbers in stock had dropped over 2004 levels. In 2003 the prefecture had 200 'small livestock raising areas' and 6000 specialized sheep raising households (defined as having 200 sheep or more in stock). The Animal Husbandry Bureau and local government were to work together to increase the number of areas specialized in sheep and sheep meat production. However, at the end of 2005, both the number of small livestock areas and households specializing in meat sheep production had dropped, partly because a major corporate driver of the specialization process in the prefecture process – the Caoyuan Xingfa Group – had experienced major logistic and financial difficulties. One area where plans were realized is in the number of breed improvement 'points' (stations), which were to increase from 500 to 1000 between the start of 2004 and the end of 2005.

The prefecture plans work their way down to lower level of government such as Lingcheng County. This county had 140,000 sheep and goats at the beginning of 2004 and planned to increase stock numbers to 250,000 by the end of 2004, to 500,000 by the end of 2005 and to 800,000 by 2008. In reality, sheep and goat numbers reached only 180,000 by the end of 2005. Plans for nearby Wongniute County were to expand its current sheep and goat numbers from 730,000 at the start of 2004 to 1 million by the end of the same year. This latter figure had been reached by the end of 2005.

In the livestock sector, a resolution of the Central Committee of the Chinese Communist Party (1998) stated that: 'With the sustainable increase of agricultural production and consumption, it is essential to pay more important attention to livestock industry, and promote its links with the farming and processing sectors'. Thus the State regards livestock industry development as a key in restructuring of the entire agricultural sector. Livestock industry development is perceived as having an important role in speeding up the 'transformation' of grain (to livestock feed), increasing rural employment opportunities, increasing farmers' incomes, promoting farming and related industry development, and stimulating rural economic development.

The Ministry of Agriculture (2001) also reports on a document drafted in 1999 entitled 'Opinion of Accelerating Livestock Development' which was approved and issued by the State Council 2001. The document states that over the next 5 to 10 years the livestock sector should be restructured by developing some livestock industries over others. Specifically the restructuring stipulated, in order of importance, that: dairy products and fine wool production should be especially targeted; beef cattle, meat sheep and meat poultry production should be promoted; and pig and poultry egg production should be developed steadily. The list was drawn up in the lead up to China's accession to the World Trade Organization based on detailed projections on the trade balance for these commodities in the period from 2005 to 2015. Findings and 'counter measures' were reported by the Ministry of Agriculture (2000).

The significance of this list and programme requires some interpretation as it has had mixed impacts in terms of tangible measures such as preferential policies and resourcing. For example, policy (and commercial) interest in dairy industry capacity has escalated dramatically, but continues to slip for fine wool production. In the case of fine wool, as discussed in Chapter 3, the market drivers encouraging the raising of sheep meat rather than fine wool both opposed and overwhelmed the policy drivers (Brown *et al.*, 2005, Chapter 8).

That the sheep and goat meat industry has been identified for promotion among the suite of other livestock industries, however, is significant. It has filtered into industry plans and signals as high level acquiescence for local government and industry actors to aggressively pursue opportunities in the industry with little risk or reprimand. As discussed below, these signals have been acted on. However, this has occurred only when these largely rhetorical 'strategic adjustment' signals have coincided with other policy measures and with other administrative and market incentives at lower levels. An awareness of the importance of local incentives is reflected in the statement of the Ministry of Agriculture (2001) that 'local government, companies, or households will adjust the structure of livestock sector according to the document and local special situation'.

Several other edicts and decrees are closely related to the notion of the 'strategic adjustment of agricultural structures'. In the Tenth 5 Year Plan (2000 to 2005), the State Economic and Trade Commission stated that 'mechanized slaughter should be implemented in all large cities across the country by the end of 2005 and the rate of mechanized slaughter should reach more than 90% in mid and small cities and county towns' (Yu, 2003). This goal has not been reached but still indicates the intention of the government.

Another government objective is flagged in the document 'Opinion of accelerating the development of agricultural processing' issued by the State Council (2003). The document states that 'over a period of development of 5 to 10 years, the agricultural processing industry should be established in a way that is conducive to the processing of "superior" agricultural products, should establish key processing enterprises and demonstration bases, technical innovation systems, complete quality and safety standards, and should increase the proportion of agricultural processing industry in gross domestic product and increase industrial adding value'. This is one of many edicts that, together, signal a shift in the policy push from production alone to processing and other parts of the industry marketing chain.

A major over-riding law that spans all aspects of the livestock sector is the China Animal Husbandry Law which was revised in December 2005 (National People's Congress, 2005). The revision strengthens provisions on breed selection processes and technical and legal standards on feed, additives and veterinary products. Most notable, however, is the emphasis on industry modernization and product quality rather than quantity. Among the measures stipulated to achieve this are for government at the county level and above to build infrastructure and to pursue larger scale rather than household-based livestock production.

## 5.1.2 *Agricultural vertical integration*

The agricultural vertical integration (*nongye chanyehua*) programme represents a more specific vehicle to pursue some of the objectives of agricultural structural adjustment. The concept of agricultural vertical integration in the Chinese context essentially aims to shorten supply chains, to develop high value market segments, to modernize agricultural industries and to develop large, vertically integrated enterprises. The Ministry of Agriculture also believes that the model will help China deal with the challenges of entry into the World Trade Organization including compliance with standards of export markets, increasing economies of scale and efficiencies (and so international competitiveness), and in developing new products and markets. For more details on the programme see Niu and Xia (2000) and Waldron *et al.* (2003, Chapter 10).

In Chinese imagery, agricultural vertical integration involves 'dragon head' organizations 'leading along' the 'length of the dragon' (the industry supply chain and its participants). The number of dragon head organizations grew from 11,824 in 1996 to 66,000 in 2000 (Niu and Xia, 2000). These comprised (in order of importance) enterprises, cooperative arrangements and specialized markets. Especially important is the relationship between the dragon head enterprises and household producers. Over the same time period, the number of vertically integrated households grew from about 20 million to 59 million (or 25% of the total agricultural households in China). Formal contracts or informal arrangements are used to 'link' or 'connect' the households to the dragon heads. The model is most developed in eastern China, followed by central and then western China. However, even in western China, the model is used as a basis to service mid to high value sheep and goat meat markets.

As with other programmes, the role of central government in the vertical integration programme is mainly to encourage, guide or coerce others to execute it. The programme, however, contains some tangible measures from central government. For example, in 2000 the Ministry of Agriculture issued an official list of 151 'preferred' agricultural and food companies and this has since been added to in two further 'rounds'. The list was drawn up to encourage the development of large enterprises better able to compete in the post World Trade Organization accession environment. About 40 of these enterprises were involved in meat production (from breeding through to meat processing, but excluding dairy, feed and aquaculture). Four of the enterprises were involved in sheep meat (Jilin Haoyue, Inner Mongolia Nailun, Caoyuan Xingfa and Henan Shuanghui). These nationally recognized dragon head enterprises are eligible to apply for special financial, tax (including exemption from tax on profits) and other support measures.

At the local level, virtually every province, city and county in China has drawn up its own list of dragon heads and developed structures to link it to household producers. Thus areas in which the sheep meat industry has gained a foothold normally have a dragon head enterprise related to sheep or sheep meat. The most common form of dragon head enterprise in the sheep meat industry is companies that produce breeding sheep (such as Hongwu, Kangda, Lukang, Santai, Dingtao Lubao and Yuncheng Dapeng). These breeding sheep enter the breeding system but are mainly for distribution to households for feeding for slaughter. That the industry is largely 'led along' by breeding companies with a focus on the very early stages of the marketing chain may be because the industry itself is in an early stage of development and still production focused.

Several notable examples exist, however, where the dragon head enterprise is a sheep abattoir or sheep meat processor (such as Caoyuan Xingfa, Haoyue, Sichuan All Star and Gaoyuan). Several companies are or planned to be fully integrated across all stages (Hongwu, Kangda and Lukang). These downstream or integrated dragon heads will become more important as the industry develops and matures. Further details on these dragon head enterprises are provided in Chapters 6 and 7. The examples of Hongwu (Box 6.4), Kangda (Box 6.5), Caoyuan Xingfa (Box 7.2) and many companies in the beef industry (see Longworth *et al.*, 2001) and certainly many others to come in the sheep industry demonstrate the risks and the problems associated with the vertical integration process in China, not only for the companies involved but also for the households that are integrated into the structures.

### 5.1.3 *Local group structures and specialization*

Local group structures feature prominently in the vertical integration programme and other sectoral or industry programmes. Local groups are seen as a 'linking mechanism' for enterprises to source agricultural inputs from households, and play a major role in improving household access to services and markets. Local groups provide a catalyst for industry growth and development and fill important functions in areas such as disease control and food safety, information and quality assurance.

Local groups are a form of organizational structure and so were also referred to in Chapter 4. They are revisited in the discussion here due to the active policy encouragement afforded to these groups. Various forms of local group structures exist including 'small areas' and associations, which are closely related to the notion of household and local-level specialization.

When the communes and brigades of the central planning era were disbanded to usher in China's reform era, extreme collectivism was replaced with extreme individualism on a household level. Throughout the 1990s in particular, local level specialization at village and township levels began to develop organically as an informal though important form of organization in Chinese agriculture. In recent years, China has sought to formalize local-level agricultural structures, but not yet to the extent of legalizing farmer cooperatives that are regarded as a potential threat to Party-state authority. Indeed, current forms of local groups are easily captured and controlled by local government and enterprises that, in turn, strategically comply with higher level dictates. Several different forms of local group structures, which often intersect, are summarized below.

Specialized 'small livestock raising areas' (*yangzhi xiaoqu*) comprise several specialized households (usually between 5 and 15) normally organized at a level below the natural village. The households participating are typically the more progressive or better resourced of the households in the natural village. They elect a head who is not necessarily a village head or party secretary. The participating households are located near to each other (and are often neighbours) and have similar or common facilities, such as livestock sheds, feed storage and treatment facilities and methane gas converters. They usually stock the same type or line of breeding ewes and cross them with genetics from the same local breeding station or artificial insemination 'point'. They also use common veterinary and feed regimes and sell through the same marketing channels.

This model has the support of central government and is being spread throughout the country. Uptake has been fastest in agricultural areas but is deemed less necessary in pastoral areas where larger scale production systems are more common and where distances between households are greater. In the semi-pastoral systems of Chifeng Prefecture in Inner Mongolia, about one third of all livestock were said to be raised in specialized small areas and there are plans to increase this to 70% by 2008 although, as mentioned in Box 5.1, these plans are unlikely to be realized. There are about 200 specialized sheep and goat-producing small areas in Chifeng in 2004 that have at least 1000 head in each. In addition, there were around 6000 specialized households which held 200 sheep or more.

Because too many areas in China were calling themselves small livestock raising areas, the Animal Husbandry Bureau at the central level tightened the definitions to: more than 200 beef or dairy cattle; more than 1000 meat sheep or goats; more than 500 fine wool sheep; and around 5000 chickens. If stock numbers in a small area exceed this range by too much, they are split into several small areas although they still maintain close relationships.

Village committees and township government and especially local Animal Husbandry Bureaus play a major role in the development of the small areas. The Animal Husbandry Bureau trains households in commercial sheep production practices, helps in the design and construction of household and common infrastructure, provides services (including breeding and veterinary services), develops marketing channels and organizes credit (especially through local credit cooperatives). In cases such as Wongniute County in Inner Mongolia, the Animal Husbandry Bureau provided significant capital (Rmb6 million) so that household members of small raising areas could obtain loans from the local credit cooperative at a subsidized rate specifically to buy sheep from a local breeding company. Policies and measures such as these alter the incentives, structures and the means by which households enter into industry activities.

Specialized villages exist at a level up from the small areas. Similarly, several specialized villages can constitute a specialized township, which can easily have a combined flock of 20,000 sheep. Sheep are raised in a limited geographical area in agricultural areas but even in pastoral areas a critical mass of homogeneous sheep can be assembled. This allows companies like Sapale in Xinjiang and Caoyuan Xingfa in Inner Mongolia to enter into purchase arrangements on a township level through township leaders who are responsible for the organization of households and livestock extension units at lower levels.

Looser and more flexible purchase arrangements, however, are more common in these specialized villages and townships. Buyers (traders, slaughter households or abattoirs) know that there is a concentration of relatively homogeneous lines of sheep in a particular small area, specialized village, or specialized township and will simply purchase from that area when required. Specialized sheep areas invariably are located close to markets that trade significant numbers of sheep and so have ready and competitive access to sheep dealers and buyers that operate out of the markets (see Chapter 6).

Specialization is not just confined to the primary production sector. Nearly every county in China with significant numbers of sheep or goats would have at least one village specialized in sheep or goat slaughtering and meat marketing. In one village in Kalaqin Banner in Chifeng City, 80% of the households were involved in livestock slaughter and meat distribution, mainly of sheep and goats. These specialized villages usually service low value sheep and goat meat markets.

As another layer in local level organization, groups of households, small areas and specialized villages often register as associations. The proliferation of local level associations has been officially endorsed and encouraged. As a result, there are hundreds of local level associations in the sheep and goat industry in China. They range from village to prefectural level in size, can be registered or unregistered, and are involved in almost any type of industry activity. Indeed, almost any form of livestock organization now uses the name 'association'. Local level associations in the sheep industry include producer groups such as small areas comprised of household producers, breeding companies where users of their stock are members, marketing companies and abattoirs. There is even an association in Inner Mongolia comprised of 10,000 livestock dealers, which was formed by the autonomous region government to improve registration and compliance with government regulations.

After the initial enthusiasm and underlying policy support for associations wanes some could be expected to fall by the wayside. Some of the more viable and well organized associations may remain in the industry and develop to play important industry functions. The associations provide a forum for members to coordinate on issues like disease control, quality control, food safety, breeding strategies, bulk input purchases and common marketing. Such functions are important to entering into and securing higher value markets including overseas markets.

All of the above mentioned forms of local groups serve to address some of the constraints of small scale, individual household based agriculture in China. The small household flock sizes can effectively be combined into larger and more uniform collective flocks. Local groups can engender a higher degree of coordination and homogeneity in the practices and type of sheep coming from local areas than would otherwise be the case if households operated individually.

Consequently, local group structures may play an important role in linking house-holds with mid and high value sheep meat markets.

### 5.1.4 The advantaged area programme

Another programme that can be classed as an industry or sector targeting policy is the 'Advantaged Area programme' (*youshiqu guihua*). This programme has been endorsed by the State Council and incorporates 11 agricultural commodities (Ministry of Agriculture, 2003b). One category combines beef cattle, meat sheep and meat goats. The place of these livestock types in the programme is addressed specifically in the document 'The Development Programme of Advantaged Areas in Beef Cattle and Meat Sheep and Goats Production' (Ministry of Agriculture, 2003a). Features of the programme are provided in Box 5.2.

The programme identifies four broad geographical and agro-climatic zones for sheep and goats,[2] namely: the Central Plains (including Henan, Shandong, Hebei and Anhui); central-east China (including Inner Mongolia and Hebei); northwest China (including Ningxia, Gansu, Qinghai and Xinjiang); and southwest China (Sichuan, Chongqing, Guizhou and Guangxi). The Central Plains sheep and goat meat belt is prioritized as the most important zone in which to pursue industry development.

Within these broad zones, the programme targets smaller administrative areas (counties or cities). The Animal Husbandry Bureau at the central level indicated that 105 areas have been chosen to participate in the programme for beef cattle and meat sheep and goats. The Ministry of Agriculture (2003a) states that there are plans to increase the number of advantaged areas to 61 for meat sheep and goats and 62 for beef cattle (although there is still uncertainty about precisely which areas will participate) and outlines criteria and the targets of the programme.

In addition to the centrally identified advantaged areas, many provinces designate their own areas. For example, there are 12 nationally determined advantaged areas for meat sheep and goats in Inner Mongolia and another 24 that are provincially determined. In Henan, 18 counties were targeted by the central government for beef cattle and meat sheep and goats and the provincial govern-ment then designated 32 counties to participate in the provincial programme.

The signals emitted from the advantaged area programme may have contrib-uted to the growth and development of the sheep and goat industry. However, few funds from central level had been tagged specifically for the programme. Instead, localities have used their own budget funds and those from other programmes – such as the Straw for Beef programme – to develop their sheep and goat meat industries in line with central government signals emitted from programmes such as the Advantaged Areas programme. As such, the programme is best seen as one part of a larger suite of policies that have overlapping aims.

---

2. For alternative regional categorizations see Brown *et al.*, 2002a.

**Box 5.2.** The 'advantaged area' programme related to the sheep and goat industry.

Centrally determined advantaged areas (counties or prefectures/cities) are selected on the criteria that they should have:

- A 'quality' breed base (with 'quality' determined by growth rates of livestock numbers and undefined meat quality characteristics)
- 200,000 head of sheep or goats, 50% of which are 'high quality'
- Advantageous resource endowments for sheep or goats (especially climate and feed)
- Established infrastructure (breeding and veterinary services and large scale slaughter plants)
- Although not formally stated, many counties chosen are active in the export trade of live cattle and sheep or goats to Hong Kong

The aims of the programme are to:

- Increase sheep or goat production by more than 38% in the 61 advantaged areas by 2007.
- Increase the proportion of 'high quality' sheep or goat meat to over 20%
- 'Standardize' production and management practices (such as homogenous lines of livestock and feed and veterinary regimes)
- Establish reputable brands of sheep and goat meat
- Replace imports and increase exports
- Develop grading and food safety systems

These aims are to be achieved through the following measures and structures:

- Breed improvement
- Pre-production systems (including the development of 'base projects' in feed production and regulation, extension, veterinary services and disease control)
- Production (sheep or goat 'bases'). These bases should develop:
  - 100 large households per county with 50 to 100 head ewes and 25 mu in land
  - 15 small livestock raising areas per county each with 500 to 2000 ewes and 250 mu of land
  - 5 feedlots per county each with over 2000 head in stock
- 20,000 silage pits per county
- Quality improvement projects (disease control and quarantine, cold storage at company level and 29 (provincial level) quality monitoring centres for breeding livestock, feed and meat
- Dragon head enterprises (centralized and accredited slaughtering, marketing or processing, companies, integrated companies, or new markets)

*Source*: (Ministry of Agriculture, 2003b).

### 5.1.5 Straw for ruminants programme

The 'Advantaged Area' programme is complementary to an earlier programme called 'Animal Production Based on Crop Residues' project, more commonly known as the 'Straw for Ruminants' programme. The Straw for Ruminants programme aims to promote the conversion of straw resources into feed (for grain saving, environmental and rural income reasons), whereas the advantaged area programme is aimed at industry commercialization and specialization. The two programmes have often been implemented in the same areas (county or prefecture/city).

The Straw for Ruminants programme was first listed in the State Agricultural Comprehensive Development Programme in 1992. From that year to 2000, 13 state level Straw for Ruminant prefectures and 380 counties were established. Of these, 269 were cattle demonstration counties and 111 were sheep and goat demonstration counties. Guo (2002) claimed that the programme played a major part in the adoption of straw ammoniation practices (more than 8 million households) and in the several-fold increases in beef, mutton and milk production. However, the the uptake and the impact of the programme are moot points. Full details and a critique of the Straw for Ruminants programme appear in Waldron *et al.* (2003, Chapter 9).

The programme is scheduled to continue to at least 2010. It is planned that ten existing prefectures and 200 existing counties will continue to participate as demonstration areas in the programme and there will be an additional 47 new prefectures and 300 new demonstration counties (Ministry of Agriculture, 2002). For a description of the way that the 'Straw for Sheep and Goats' programme will be extended in Wuyuan County in Inner Mongolia see Wang and Zhang (2002).

## 5.2 Social and environmental policies

The sectoral and industry policies discussed above are closely related to social and environmental policies discussed in this section. Indeed, the attempt to achieve multiple objectives is a feature of policy making in China. Industry, social and environmental policies tend to be top down and interventionist in nature in China.

### 5.2.1 Poverty alleviation

China's poverty alleviation programme has been redefined several times since 1978. Economic reforms in the early 1980s lifted hundreds of millions of households out of poverty and efforts shifted to supplying the 'basic needs' of those still in poverty. Following the move towards a 'pro growth' strategy, poverty alleviation funds were channelled to households as bank or credit cooperative loans but were plagued by defaults. Emphasis then turned toward financing the development of local enterprises – including those involved in agriculture – but concerns arose as to the degree that this could benefit poor households (Rozelle *et al.*, 1998). In recent years, considerable poverty alleviation funding has been made available to larger households to act as a model for small, poorer households.

By 2005, the targets of China's poverty alleviation programme have become a more sophisticated mix of all those mentioned above. Local governments largely decided the relative weight on the different targets and have a high degree of discretion over the use of the funds which comes from central, provincial and local sources. Agriculture is a major vehicle for delivery of poverty alleviation funds. In many poor, rural, remote areas of China, options are often confined to the ruminant livestock sector and poverty alleviation efforts have a strong industry focus.

About 50 – or one half – of the counties in Inner Mongolia are declared as poverty stricken. Inner Mongolia spends Rmb100 million on poverty alleviation every year, most of which is used for livestock production, especially in the dairy, sheep and goat industries.[3] In many areas in Inner Mongolia, such as Wongniute County, sheep production is the single biggest industry. Wongniute receives about 50% of its gross domestic product from agriculture, of which 50% is from livestock. Within the livestock sector, about 20% of households are specialized in meat sheep production, and 15% in wool sheep.

This type of economic structure is common throughout the pastoral region, but less so in other areas of China where households have a wider range of economic alternatives. For example, in Heze Prefecture in Shandong Province, the production value of livestock in total agriculture ranges between 23% and 30%. Sheep and cattle production each make up about 18% of the livestock production value. However, these industries are seen as an important way of lifting households out of poverty in Heze's two nationally declared and three provincially declared poverty counties.

In areas that have prioritized development of the sheep industry, sheep breeding activities are seen as an important means of aiding households, including poverty-stricken households. The funding can be used in various ways. Sheep breeding stations such as the Santai Company (Ningcheng County, Chifeng Prefecture of Inner Mongolia) and the Shan County Sheep Breeding Farm in Liangshan County (Heze Prefecture in Shandong) were partly or fully invested through poverty alleviation funds.

Breeding stations of all ownership types – state run, shareholder, privately owned – can access poverty alleviation funds for activities that link with households. Poverty alleviation funds are commonly used to facilitate household sheep purchases from breeding stations under various schemes. The funds are used to subsidize loans (in the form of low interest repayments or interest waivers) from local banks or credit cooperatives that are taken out by households for the express purpose of purchasing (female) sheep from the breeding station. The household is responsible for repaying the loans mainly from the proceeds of sales of offspring. Alternatively, the loan can often be paid back by selling lambs back to the breeding station itself. Companies such as Lukang (in Wongniute County in Inner Mongolia) involve households in the feeding of male lambs to slaughter age with the breed station then marketing the sheep as one homogeneous mob to abattoirs. Some companies such as Hongwu have their own abattoirs to slaughter the sheep. More commonly, female lambs are sold (or repaid) back to the breeding station to grow the overall breeding flock of the company, which are then sent out to other households.

Many projects are based on the Small Tailed Han sheep breed because of their high levels of fecundity (averaging nine lambs every 2 years) and relatively high

---

3. This Rmb100 million does not include matching funds from other levels of government or programmes involving micro credit and interest subsidization.

live weights. However, the low quality meat from this breed of sheep combined with the rapid growth rate in sheep numbers means that the suitability of these schemes in markets in the future needs to be carefully assessed on an ongoing basis. Meat sheep production is perceived as a good livestock activity for lifting households out of poverty in China because sheep are less prone to disease and less technically demanding to manage than many other livestock types. Some poverty alleviation activities also target household housing and feed infrastructure as a means of improving sheep production practices and reducing risks to households.

The Shan County Sheep Breeding Farm in Shandong Province illustrates how livestock are used in poverty alleviation programmes in China. Image 5.1 shows the structure and the impact of the programme. The first (left hand) column shows the year of the programme, the second column shows the increase in breeding sheep numbers in poverty stricken households (in the townships), the third column shows the increase in the core breeding flock of the Shan County breeding farm, while the fourth column shows the total increase in the number of sheep in the programme. These figures are calculated on the basis that 1000 breeding ewes are invested in the breeding programme in 2000, each of which produces three lambs per year, which is possible for highly productive Small Tailed Han sheep. Half of these offspring are males and half are females. In the first year, the households are obliged to pass on the same number of sheep

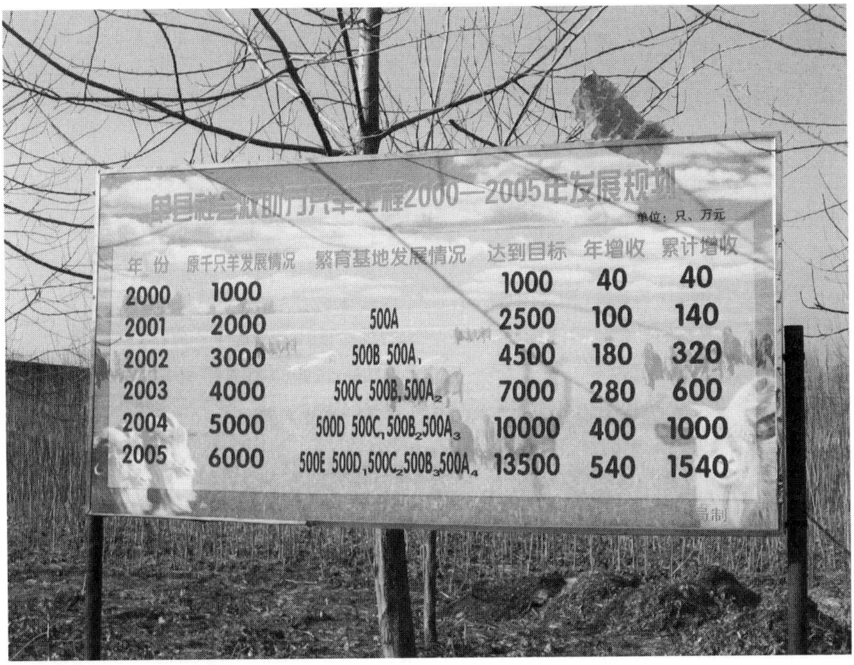

**Image 5.1.** Planned flock structure of the Shan County sheep breeding station poverty alleviation programme.

that they received (1000) to the next group of poverty stricken households. In addition, every year they are obliged to return half this number (500) back to the Shan County breeding station. The households keep the original sheep they received (1000 head). This leads to the cumulative total of all sheep in the programme (fourth column). Each of these sheep are valued at Rmb400 to give (in units of Rmb10,000) the annual values (fifth column) and the cumulative value of sheep over the programme (sixth column). On this basis, officials in the programme estimate that an investment of 1000 sheep in the year 2000 leads to 13,500 sheep in 2005 worth Rmb5.4 million. These figures do not reflect the value of the male sheep (that are sold as slaughter sheep), or the extra females that are retained by households after their initial first year obligations, which can lead to a much higher growth in sheep numbers.

Image 5.2 shows the way that sheep in the programme are distributed between households in 20 different townships in Shan County. The top box in each of the townships represents the total number of sheep planned to be distributed to each township (to total 13,500 sheep) while the bottom box are the numbers that had actually been sent out by the end of 2004.

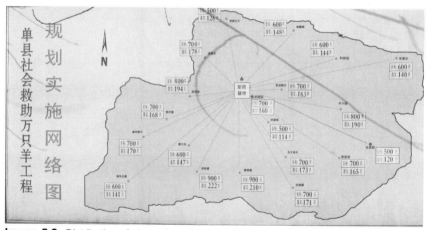

**Image 5.2.** Distribution of sheep from the Shan County sheep breeding station to poverty stricken households in 20 townships.

### 5.2.2 Grassland protection measures

Although Chapter 2 outlined the spatial shift in sheep numbers in China, the pastoral region still accounts for a significant proportion of meat sheep numbers. However, major environmental problems in the form of grassland degradation are undermining the basis of sheep production in the region. Longworth and Williamson (1993) detail the cycle of increasing human populations, higher grazing pressures, degrading grasslands and reduced grazing income. China has belatedly begun to address the massive problem of grassland degradation through a raft of measures. One aspect of the Develop the West programme of the late 1990s relates to environmental protection. Then in 2002, the State Council promulgated a document titled 'Opinions on Strengthening Grassland Protection and Development', while a new Grassland Law was passed by the People's Congress and came into effect on 1 March, 2003.

More radically, in 2003 China officially launched the 'Reduce livestock, return the grasslands programme'.[4] The vast majority of the attention and the resources in the programme have been targeted at infrastructure and increasing the productivity of the grasslands, especially though fencing and pasture improvement. The long term intent is to increase the carrying capacity of the grasslands.

In the shorter term, other measures have been taken to reduce pressure on the grasslands. These include compensation for cultivating less land in sensitive areas of the grasslands (as part of the 'Grain for Green' programme). The main measure is to facilitate the transition from extensive grazing (on pastures) to intensive feeding (pen feeding). Implementation of the 'Reduce livestock, return the grasslands' programme has varied in different areas, depending on agro-climatic conditions and the condition of grasslands. For example, as of 2006 all counties in Chifeng City were subject to a total grazing ban. This notionally means that grass, forage and grain must be cut and carried to livestock held in pens. In other parts of Inner Mongolia, grasslands can be grazed only for a few months of the year, namely in late summer after the grasslands have recovered from winter and grown throughout spring. In other parts of the pastoral regions, however, the policy has not been applied at all.

Although the grazing ban appears to be a drastic policy measure, there are several factors that reduce its impact. The variability in programmes and policy implementation reflects the diversity of the grasslands, the autonomy delegated to local authorities and the limited resources attached to the programmes. Programmes such as the 'Reduce livestock, return the grasslands' are undertaken on a trial basis and are periodically reviewed. Furthermore, the logistics of policing such a large area make complete grazing bans or stocking limits difficult to enforce, especially as the programme has generally decreased incomes of sheep producers.

Grasslands policies, regulations and programmes have and will continue to impact on meat sheep production in western regions. Although not evident in the macro (province) level statistics, the measures have impacted on livestock numbers in some areas. For example, Ningcheng County in Chifeng City has experienced a fall in sheep and goat numbers from 270,000 head in 2001 to 140,000 head in 2004 as a result of the grassland regulations. Households either did not have enough self produced feed or lacked the economic incentives to buy in feed to feed sheep in pens for the whole year.

---

4. This is known as *tuimu huancao* programme. An earlier and similar programme is the Beijing-Tianjin Desertification project which incorporates a vast area of grasslands in northern China that blows sand into the two cities. More details on China's grasslands programmes are reported in Brown *et al.*, 2007.

Environmental considerations and regulations will also impact on the way that sheep and grasslands are managed in the pastoral areas of China. An increase in intensive feeding practices has the potential to increase the coordination of veterinary, breeding and feeding regimes and to increase the coordination of the marketing of outputs. It may also encourage households to turn off livestock at a younger age to avoid carrying stock into longer and more expensive feeding periods. In pastoral areas, officials and companies (such as Caoyuan Xingfa) encourage households to finish slaughter lambs in the allowed grazing period from July to September. Some county officials also claim that the new regulations will reduce goat numbers relative to sheep numbers, as sheep respond better to shed feeding and because goats are more destructive to the grasslands. For further analysis of this issues see Bai (2002).

## 5.3 Market support services

China has placed increased emphasis in recent years on the development of market support services for agricultural industries, including food safety standards, grading and information. In general, however, these systems remain underdeveloped for a number of reasons. First, sectoral or industry or interventionist policies discussed above are emphasized more strongly as a means of pursuing industry development. Second, industries such as sheep meat that are at an early stage of development may not warrant a sophisticated set of market systems. Third, China is still in the process of developing the necessary institutional structures to deliver industry services. The discussion below highlights the low level of market support services in the sheep meat industry, but also the way in which these systems are likely to develop into the future. Systems that improve the accuracy of the market signals that industry participants respond to are undoubtedly of interest to the government. However, the fragmented nature of the industry and the diverse array of benefits and costs from the system entail difficulties in developing and implementing cost effective industry-wide schemes.

### 5.3.1 Food safety standards

Over the post reform era, China has implemented a raft of laws and regulations relating to food quality, safety and sanitation. A wide consensus exists, however, that these are often outdated, uncoordinated, and not monitored effectively. As a consequence, consumers have little confidence in China's food quality system (see, for example, *People's Daily*, 2004). Problems associated with the inspection of feedstuff, animal diseases, slaughter facilities and meat for the beef industry are discussed in detail in Waldron *et al.* (2003, Chapter 13), and similar issues are experienced in the sheep and goat meat industries. The difficulties associated with enforcing hygiene standards in industries dominated by small scale producers, household slaughtering and a fragmented meat distribution system are discussed in Brown *et al.* (2002b).

Given the inadequacy of the public systems, various other food safety systems have been developed. These are most applicable to higher grade products. Indeed, as outlined in Chapter 3, much of the premium for sheep and goat meat is related to the delivery of safety assured product.

One set of standards for the sheep meat industry is the Green Foods standards. The Green Food certification scheme is run by the China Green Food Development Centre, a service centre under the Ministry of Agriculture. Green Food offices operate down to province levels and other related bodies include the China Green Food Association and the Green Food Consumer Network. Different grades (A or AA) are applied depending on practices employed during production and processing, including hygiene.[5]

At the beginning of 2003, China had 1929 companies using Green Food labels of which 22 companies produce or market sheep meat products. With one exception, all of these are from the pastoral areas of Xinjiang, Qinghai, Shanxi and Inner Mongolia. Examples include the Caoyuan Xingfa Group, Gaoyuan Green Food Development Corporation of Qinghai Meat Group and the Qinghai Datong Muslim Meat Company. Because sheep meat has traditionally – and to a large extent still is – associated with extensive pastoral systems, there would appear to be significant scope to expand the market acceptance of sheep meat by building the association between sheep meat and Green Foods in the minds of consumers.

An array of other schemes has also been established to alleviate consumer concerns about food safety. The 'safety foods' (*wugonghai shipin*) system is administered by the Ministry of Agriculture and is applied to foods that meet national food standards. The Ministry of Agriculture also runs an 'Organic Food' (*youji shipin*) system. Another system called 'healthy foods' (*baojian shipin*) is operated by the National Food and Drug Administration Bureau under the Ministry of Health. A less formal scheme is the 'trustworthy meat' (*fangxinrou*) established under the 'Vegetable Basket' programme. The background and continued association of sheep meat as a food for Muslim minorities, means that many sheep meat products produced using Halal practices are endorsed by the Islamic Association. Many of these schemes are overseen by the General Administration of Quality Supervision, Inspection and Quarantine.

Another very important *de facto* form of quality assurance is company and product branding and reputations. This form of branding arises because consumers generally have little confidence in the application of public standards especially as they are applied to small scale slaughter households and private meat distributors in China. Large companies and state owned companies are thought to be better managed and monitored. The products of many of these companies are commonly certified by at least one of the schemes discussed above which are designed predominantly for large companies. For instance the Bangjie

---

5. Details on the China Green Food system are available at http://www.greenfood.org.cn (in Chinese).

company in Henan had several forms of accreditation including 'safety food', ISO accreditation and a 'Certification of Products Conformity'.

### 5.3.2 Grading systems

Apart from food standards, food grading systems aim to identify degrees of product quality. Formal, extensive grading systems do not exist in China for any type of meat (China Meat Association, personal communication, 2004). There are no widely recognized public grading systems that use objective criteria for sheep meat in China. Furthermore there is little underlying demand for such systems for the majority of the sheep meat trade in China, which is low value in nature, and sold on wet markets in generic, undifferentiated lumps. In general, customers are not concerned about the meat quality characteristics of sheep meat, especially Western notions of 'quality', for many of the dishes for which it is prepared.

Nevertheless, rudimentary and informal forms of sheep meat grading are commonly used in China especially in the mid and high value markets. The informal systems are based on the following factors:[6]

- *Types of cuts.* Even in low value wet markets, differentiation between goat and sheep meat usually occurs. Some sheep meat cuts – such as fillet and hindquarter meat – are sold as separate cuts, as is bone in meat from the neck, ribs, shank and backbone. As discussed in Chapter 7, price differentials between cuts of sheep meat can arise in wholesale markets, supermarkets and higher value restaurants.
- *Age of the animal slaughtered.* From a low base, consumers are beginning to recognize the difference between lamb and mutton, and that slaughter age affects characteristics such as tenderness. This is partly due to marketing campaigns by companies such as Caoyuan Xingfa for products such as the '180 day' and 'current year' lamb. Chinese preferences with regard to characteristics such as flavour and tenderness, however, often differ to western preferences partly because of different cooking and eating methods.
- *Source of the sheep.* Some parts of the pastoral area (such as western Inner Mongolia) are recognized as producing higher quality sheep meat than other (especially agricultural) areas. This is often emphasized in marketing and packaging.
- *Number of cuts.* Much of the sheep meat trade is conducted based on the number of times the carcass is 'divided'. This can range from none (for a whole carcass), to one (half carcasses), to eight cuts (where specific cuts are differentiated). A positive relationship exists between the number of times the carcass is divided and price due to the butchering costs involved and the practice of averaging price across cuts. For export orders and the domestic restaurant trade, customers dictate the number of cuts.

---

6. Consumers in some parts of China – such as Inner Mongolia – are much more discerning and educated about sheep meat than some other areas of China where sheep meat is a more recent addition to the diet.

- *Type of cuts.* In supermarkets and also in some wholesale and retail markets, some stalls sell particular cuts of meat.

The implementation of grading systems for meat has the potential to address various marketing inefficiencies in the area of pricing accuracy but is a vexed issue not only for China but also in countries with more developed livestock sectors. Even with advanced testing and monitoring processes and with more intensive and higher value livestock industries, the costs of implementing grading systems are high. The fragmented nature of China's meat industry and the problems in monitoring are likely to make unit costs of grading even higher. The high costs must be reconciled against benefits which are minimal in the low value market segments. Even in the high value market segments, major companies see their own private branding, product description and grading systems as a source of differentiation and competitive advantage and are therefore unlikely to participate in a public grading system. While a public grading system may be warranted in mid value market segments (Waldron *et al.*, 2003), widespread adoption will take some time and further industry development for the benefits to exceed the costs.

Consumer protection regulations such as the Product Quality Law of 1993 exist to encourage product description to reflect the actual product. The degree to which this is the case in China is largely determined by the knowledge of the customers about meat and their relationship with the vendors, rather than in objective labelling in packing. For more anonymous trading over long distances, the reputation of the companies is an important means of reducing product risk. Even in this case, however, misrepresentation can occur. Sheep meat for the hot pot trade is commonly sold in rolls where it is difficult to differentiate between cuts of mutton and lamb, let alone the cuts in the packages and the place of production. The source of the sheep meat is sometimes misrepresented. A recent survey of 13 cities conducted by the State Administration for Industry and Commerce found that only 38 of 67 samples taken passed national standards (Minter Ellison, 2005). The main problem, especially pronounced in beef and sheep meat, was excessive water content, due to the injection of water into the meat to make it look juicy and increase the weight of the product.

### 5.3.3 Market reporting

China has ambitions to develop its market reporting system for a large number of agricultural products. However, the absence of an objective and widely accepted grading system for sheep meat in China has precluded the development of a price reporting system of sufficient level of disaggregation to be useful to industry participants. That is, it is not possible to collect disaggregated price information for different grades and types of sheep meat if there is no widely accepted and objective means of differentiating between different grades and types of sheep meat. Consequently, price information is collected only for generic sheep and goat meat combined.

As discussed in Chapter 3, official price information for sheep and goat meat (combined) provides a broad indication of price movements over time (month) and price differentials over space (to provincial levels). Data are collected from observation points at markets throughout China and reported through various government reports, newspapers and industry magazines. These data may arguably be useful for actors in the low value segments of the industry if it was disseminated more widely to, for example, household sheep and sheep meat producers and local dealers. However, it is of limited use for domestic participants in the mid or high value sheep and goat meat sectors, or for exporters to China. In the absence of a detailed national official market reporting system, other less comprehensive systems have developed which are based on particular wholesale markets that report on the internet.

## 5.4 Trade policies

As is the case with agricultural policies in many developed countries, trade policies are closely connected with domestic policies. In particular, many domestic policies are designed to improve China's competitive position on an international level, to compete with and to replace sheep meat imports and to promote sheep meat exports. Thus domestic industry policies have a large bearing on the conduct of trade, perhaps more so than does trade policy itself. This is particularly the case given the trade liberalization measures that have been undertaken in various multilateral agreements and bilateral agreements in recent years. Even in the context of trade liberalization, however, China's trade regime also provides scope for the use of several forms of non-tariff barriers.

### 5.4.1 Sheep meat imports

The institutional and regulatory environment in which the sheep meat trade takes place has begun to consolidate after years of significant change. The changes have impacted on the structure and the corporate actors in both the import and export sectors. In terms of government institutions, in 1998 the Department of Entry-Exit Inspection and Quarantine under the General Administration of Quality Supervision, Inspection and Quarantine took charge from the Ministry of Agriculture of the inspection of imported foods including meat, for product description, quality and hygiene. Tariffs are collected by China Customs, which is also responsible for investigating smuggling.

Various trade agreements have or will reduce the importance of tariffs as an instrument of regulating trade. Accession to the World Trade Organization in 2001 committed China to reducing import tariffs on most categories of fresh/ chilled or frozen sheep meat and offal as shown in Table 5.1. Only carcasses and half carcasses of sheep (both in the fresh/chilled and frozen forms) will not see a reduction in tariff rates, possibly because the low level of transformation (butchering) and processing that these products are subjected to may be perceived to make them more cost competitive with domestic product. In addition to multilateral agreements, there are reports that Australia (and other countries) will seek zero import tariff rates for various meat products in bilateral Free Trade Agreements with China.

The meat trade is conducted by an increasingly well organized and informed import and export sector. On the import side, China has dismantled import monopolies in a range of industries, including meat. Any Chinese company that meets capital registration and legal status criteria can be licensed to import meat. Chinese meat importers have built up strong contacts and knowledge in the industry. In addition, foreign companies can now register to import and distribute commodities including meat as set out in the 'Guide on Foreign Companies

**Table 5.1.** Change in import tariffs for sheep, sheep meat and sheep offal under agreements associated with China's accession to the World Trade Organization.

| HS Code | Article Description | General (%) | Most Favoured Nation status (%) | | | | | |
|---|---|---|---|---|---|---|---|---|
| | | | 2000 | 2001 | 2002 | 2003 | 2004 | 2005–2010 |
| Live sheep and goats | | | | | | | | |
| 0104 | Pure bred breeding sheep | 0 | 0 | 0 | 0 | 0 | 0 | 0 |
| 0104 | Others (non breeding) | 50 | 10 | 10 | 10 | 10 | 10 | 10 |
| Meat of sheep or goat, fresh, chilled or frozen | | | | | | | | |
| 02041000 | Carcasses and half carcasses of lamb, fresh or chilled | 70 | 23 | 19.8 | 18.2 | 16.6 | 15 | 15 |
| 02042100 | Carcasses and half carcasses of sheep, fresh or chilled | 70 | 23 | 23 | 23 | 23 | 23 | 23 |
| 02042200 | Bone-in cuts of sheep meat, fresh or chilled | 70 | 23 | 19.8 | 18.2 | 16.6 | 15 | 15 |
| 02042300 | Bone-out cuts of sheep meat, fresh or chilled | 70 | 23 | 19.8 | 18.2 | 16.6 | 15 | 15 |
| 02043000 | Carcasses and half carcasses of lamb, frozen | 70 | 23 | 19.8 | 18.2 | 16.6 | 15 | 15 |
| 02044100 | Carcasses and half carcasses of sheep, frozen | 70 | 23 | 23 | 23 | 23 | 23 | 23 |
| 02044200 | Bone-in cuts of sheep meat, frozen | 70 | 23 | 18.6 | 16.4 | 14.2 | 12 | 12 |
| 02044300 | Bone-out cuts of sheep meat, frozen | 70 | 23 | 19.8 | 18.2 | 16.6 | 15 | 15 |
| 02045000 | Goat meat, fresh, chilled or frozen | 70 | 23 | 21.8 | 21.2 | 20.6 | 20 | 20 |
| Offal of sheep and goats | | | | | | | | |
| 02068000 | Offal, fresh or chilled | 70 | 20 | 20 | 20 | 20 | 20 | 20 |
| 02069000 | Offal, frozen | 70 | 20 | 19.2 | 18.8 | 18.4 | 18 | 18 |

*Source*: Document provided by the Ministry of Agriculture.

Investment in China' (National Development and Reform Commission, 2002). Application and registration procedures are essentially the same as that of a Chinese company.

All exporters have been able to and still can supply meat to deluxe hotels, the diplomatic service, re-exporters and the manufacturing sector. However, with China's accession to the World Trade Organization and the establishment of various bilateral quarantine and health protocols, access to the broader Chinese market is currently limited to certified exporters. The certification body is the Department of Registration Management, within the State Administration for Certification and Accreditation, under the General Administration of Quality Supervision, Inspection and Quarantine. Trade and other officials of many countries have argued that the number of establishments certified to export to China has been restricted as a means of restricting meat imports. In the case of Australia, numbers were tightly restricted to three establishments (two for beef and one for sheep meat) but were increased in stages to reach 45 by 2005. Currently these plants must slaughter, bone and package in one integrated establishment. However, signs have emerged that independent plants may also be certified to export to China provided that they source from one of these 45 integrated establishments.

China has also restricted the supply of sheep and goat offal to China, including tripe from Australia that can be subject to stringent micro testing. Some overseas interests claim this to be a form of non-tariff barrier and have been forced to export tripe (in large quantities) through an exemption category. Indeed, Ministry of Agriculture officials openly express concern about the impact that large volumes of imported offal (which is a relatively low value commodity in many western countries and not subject to high levels of transformation) might have on the domestic industry. However, some of the issues associated with tripe imports may be resolved in the context of bilateral agreements and protocols.

Importers must obtain permits to import meat shipments. The import permits specify the source of the meat (certified establishment), product types (including primal cut description) and volumes to be imported (tonnage). While this process has become increasingly manageable, the length of time for processing the permits – often more than a month – can restrict the ability of traders to take advantage of short term market opportunities. There have been reports of shipments being rejected or held up by Chinese authorities because the product description (primal cuts) on the import permit did not match the labels on the meat (which must be labelled in dual languages), and also due to Listeria concerns (which were not able to be verified through Australian tests). Inspection of shipments is done on a random basis and there is zero tolerance for microbiological contamination by organisms such as *E. coli* and *Salmonella*.

China's accession to the World Trade Organization required recognition of the World Trade Organization Agreement on Sanitary and Phytosanitary Measures. These measures state that all animal, plant and human health import requirements must be based on scientific grounds. Additional bilateral agreements have also been established, including the 'Protocol between the General Administration of Quality Supervision Inspection and Quarantine of the People's Republic of China and the Australian Department of Agriculture, Fisheries and Forestry on Quarantine and Veterinary Sanitary Conditions of Meat from Sheep or Goats to be Exported from Australia to China'. China's signing of these formal agreements represents a first step for improved access to the Chinese market. However, addressing China's political approach to trade management on an industry-by-industry or sector-by-sector basis will require prolonged negotiations and ongoing communication which will be aided by an understanding of the Chinese industry and issues faced by Chinese negotiators.

### 5.4.2 Sheep and genetic imports

As indicated in Table 5.1, tariffs on 'other' (slaughter) livestock have been reduced but still exceed that for breeding livestock. China is more permissive on the import of breeding livestock to improve China's domestic flock. As outlined in Table 5.1, breeding stock are imported into China tariff free. There are a range of other protocols on the import of livestock that are often deemed unscientific in nature (although strictly speaking these also apply to breeding livestock). For example, rather than follow the Australian vector line for blue tongue, China bans imports of most livestock from states north of Victoria.

At the same time, Chinese policy makers are concerned about the possibility that imported genetic material may carry diseases or breed unsuitable traits into the Chinese flock. Consequently, China has developed a series of institutions, regulations and procedures for the important of genetic materials, including breeding sheep. The Animal Husbandry Bureau signs general protocols for the import of livestock and is integral to the approval process for particular orders.

**Box 5.3.** Procedures for importing breeding sheep and genetic material.

- Importers complete an application form including the reasons for the import. The province Animal Husbandry Bureau forwards the application to the Animal Husbandry Department at central level for approval.
- A more detailed plan is then prepared covering: types, quantity, sex, country of origin, date and ports of entry, and number of batches.
- Details on the source of the capital and bank credit certificate are shown, along with the supply agreement and a letter of intent of the foreign agency.
- A list of experts from China is drawn up who will travel overseas to select the breeding sheep or genetic material. The foreign sheep breed association or society provides the pedigree certificates. For the breeding livestock to be eligible for duty free import, these certificates are now required to extend back three generations.
- The breeders or genetic material are then subject to quarantine at the port under the supervision of the Department of Animal Quarantine.

*Source*: Documents provided by the Ministry of Agriculture.

**Box 5.4.** Quarantine and inspection of imported breeding and live animals.

According to the regulations of 'Quarantine Law for the Entry and Exit of Animals and Plants of the People's Republic of China' (1992), imported animals, embryo, semen and other genetic materials are subject to the following quarantine procedures:

- Prior to import, animal quarantine departments or veterinary administration departments of both governments need to sign a quarantine protocol for imported animals and genetic materials.

- Importers bring forward an application to the State Inspection and Quarantine Department to undergo quarantine examination and approval procedures, and a quarantine licence is then issued.

- Importers then request quarantine inspection at the port. At port, quarantine officials check the 'Certification of Animal Quarantine' issued by the quarantine or veterinary administration department of the exporting country, inspect the consignment and sterilize areas affected by animals. Quarantine staff will then authorize the movement of livestock and genetic materials to appointed sites for further isolation quarantine.

- Isolation quarantine will then take place at specified sites at selected ports. For horses, cattle, sheep, goats and pigs, these are located in Beijing, Tianjin, Shanghai and Guangzhou, although other sites can be approved by the State Department of Inspection and Quarantine. During the quarantine period (45 days for large and mid-sized animals and 30 days for small animals like sheep), quarantine officials at the port undertake clinical inspection, sampling and laboratory inspection.

- On completion of the quarantine period, the Department of Inspection and Quarantine at the port fills out a 'Certification of Animal Quarantine' and related papers which allows the livestock and genetic materials to 'enter' China. The Department of Inspection and Quarantine can authorize animals suffering from infectious diseases and verminosis to be returned (to the country of origin) or destroyed according to the relevant provisions and protocols of the Ministry of Agriculture.

However, a different agency – the Department of Inspection and Quarantine under the General Administration of Quality Supervision, Inspection and Quarantine – oversees agreements relating to specific orders and shipments.

Several sets of regulations govern the import of breeding sheep and genetic material. These include 'Regulations on Breeding Livestock and Poultry Administration' issued by the State Council in 1994, and the 'Detailed Implementation Rules of Regulations on Breeding Livestock and Poultry Administration' issued by the Ministry of Agriculture in 1998. Provincial agricultural departments also have detailed implementation rules. Under the 'Detailed Implementation Rules of Regulations on Breeding Livestock and Poultry Administration' issued by the Ministry of Agriculture in 1998, there are restrictions on the breeds of livestock that can (and can not) be imported and exported. The Ministry of Agriculture has prepared the list of breeds and executes the programme. Other detailed procedures for import to China, quarantine and inspection of breeding stock and genetic material are outlined in Box 5.3 and Box 5.4.

# 6

# Livestock sector developments

Previous chapters have illustrated the recent rapid expansion of the Chinese sheep meat industry and argued that this growth has been the result of a potent mix of market, institutional and policy drivers. As will be demonstrated in this chapter and the next, this mix of factors has driven enormous changes in agribusiness structures. Different drivers have had different impacts on different parts of the marketing chain. In particular, most institutional and policy attention has been directed toward the early stages of the marketing chain, especially breeding and sheep production. Thus analysis of agribusiness aspects of the industry begins in this chapter with sheep breeding, production and marketing. Chapter 7 continues the discussion with a focus on downstream sheep meat sectors.

## 6.1 Breeding

Within Chinese livestock industries, the breeding sector is seen as the first step and the base from which the rest of the industry is built. Planners and participants in the sector tend to emphasize the technical and physical attributes of the genetic base. However, these attributes do not necessarily bear a close relationship to the product attributes either in demand from downstream actors or that are likely to maximize long term returns. Because breeding activities have a long term impact on the quantity and quality of product (sheep meat) produced, analysis of the sector can provide some insights into the future direction of the industry. This section examines the breeding sector and its development in terms of the sheep breeds in China, breeding stations and structures in China, and the conduct of breeding activities as an agribusiness activity.

### 6.1.1 Breeds

The Ministry of Agriculture directs China's breeding programme on several basic principles. The ultimate goal is to raise the productivity of sheep using introduced breeds to improve local breeds. Pure bred flocks are to be used as the 'base' for the programme with improvement occurring through cross breeding. To understand the nature and the driving factors behind this breeding programme, some features of China's sheep genetic resources need to be outlined.

Several studies report on China's sheep breeding resources. One of the most recent and comprehensive is entitled *Domestic Animal Genetic Resources in China* (Ministry of Agriculture, 2003c).[1] The study reported that China had 50 registered breeds of sheep of which 31 were native breeds, with 20 originating from northwest China. China has bred another nine 'developed' breeds, which are Merino crosses and reflect China's long history in breeding for fine wool production. The fine wool sheep breeding programme has been achieved through the introduction of the Australian Merino which is one of only ten sheep breeds introduced from overseas. The other nine are meat sheep breeds and include Charolais, Corriedale, Lincoln, Romney, German Merino, Suffolk, Poll Dorset and Texel. Unlike the Australian Merinos, China has access to both purebred meat sheep ewes and rams. China imported a total of 14,628 breeding sheep between 1997 and 2005, of which more than 80% came from Australia and nearly 20% from New Zealand. As discussed below, however, larger numbers of embryos are imported.

The significant number of sheep breeds and crosses in China precludes a comprehensive examination of Chinese sheep genetics. However, fieldwork revealed some trends in the development of major meat sheep breeds. Various local sheep breeds exist in Inner Mongolia (including Ujumqin, Sunite and Helinge'er) but the most important is the Mongolian breed of which there were 20 million head in China in 1986. This fat-tailed breed is well adapted to the harsh conditions of northern China but has relatively low growth rates and has traditionally been slaughtered at a relatively old age.[2] The high fat cover and strong taste of the meat mean they are well suited to traditional Mongolian dishes. They are also highly sought after in the broader Chinese sheep meat market. Nearly all hot pot restaurants source – or claim to source – sheep meat from Mongolian breed sheep from Inner Mongolia.

A major feature in China's sheep breed improvement programme in recent years has been cross-breeding with Small Tailed Han sheep, which originate from Shandong (see Image 6.1).[3] Officials in Shandong estimated that in 2003

---

1. Other publications include Editorial Board on the Breeds of Domestic Animal and Poultry in China (1986) which details China's sheep and goat breeds, including estimates of numbers by breed type. A large number of other publications provide information on the characteristics of local and introduced sheep breeds in China, many of which are listed on http://www.chinasheep.com. The China Sheep Association has also produced a handbook on native and introduced breeds (China Sheep Association, no date-b).
2. Outstanding examples of the Mongolian breed in Alashan in Inner Mongolia reached 47 kg for rams and 32 kg for ewes. The bone-in dressing rate was 47% to 52%, and 35% bone out. Lambs can be slaughtered at 5 to 7 months of age at a liveweight of 13 to 18 kg and a bone-in dressing percentage of about 40%.
3. There are seven 'production bases' (counties) in Shandong where the Small Tailed Han breed is preserved. These are in Heze Prefecture (Yuncheng, Juye and Zhuancheng counties), Jining Prefecture (Liangshan and Jiacheng counties) and Taiyang Prefecture (Dongping County). The breed is certified by the Shandong Livestock and Poultry Breed Committee.

the province had sold out a total of about 1 million Small Tailed Han sheep, mainly for breeding purposes, and that these genetics had been infused into about 10 million sheep in 20 provinces. Officials in Inner Mongolia estimated that by 2004 the autonomous region had imported 50,000 to 60,000 Small Tailed Han sheep for breeding purposes.

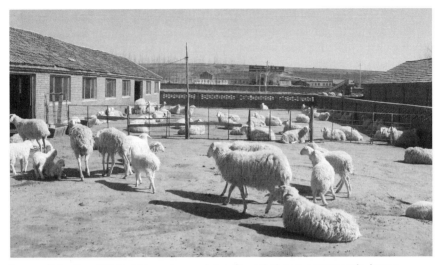

**Image 6.1.** Small Tailed Han sheep at the Santai sheep company in Inner Mongolia. These large and highly productive sheep have become an important part of China's meat sheep breeding programme. Breeding stations in Inner Mongolia have brick shedding facilities to protect stock from harsh winters.

Industry officials and participants are attracted to the very high fecundity and growth characteristics of the breed, as outlined in Box 6.1.[4] The rapid dissemination of the breed has been a major contributor to the very high growth rates of the industry and enables industry officials to set ambitious production targets. However, widespread concerns have emerged about the poor eating quality of the breed, particularly in Inner Mongolia which aims to supply higher value sheep meat markets.[5] Various cross-breeding programmes have sought to address a decline in eating quality through cross-breeding programmes with both local and introduced breeds such as Poll Dorsets.

The trend toward developing highly productive meat sheep breeds was especially pronounced in eastern parts of Inner Mongolia which have large tracts of semi-pastoral land, intensive feeding systems and sheep housing infrastructure. For example, Chifeng Prefecture is improving its local sheep herd with Small Tailed Han sheep and imported breeds on the basis that: local breeds are well

---

4. For further details on the breed see He (2002).
5. This perception is debated by Zeng *et al.* (2000).

adapted to local conditions and the meat suits traditional Mongolian dishes; Small Tailed Han sheep are highly productive; and crossings with imported breeds mature early and offset the negative meat quality traits of Small Tailed Han sheep.

Despite the significant number of sheep breeds in China, no formal breed societies operate as is common in many countries with developed livestock industries and that also notionally exist in the beef cattle industry in China. Instead, some local level associations (such as for Small Tailed Han sheep) exist to help coordinate breeding companies and households in their early stages of development, while livestock certification and performance recording and testing is notionally undertaken by the local Animal Husbandry Bureau.

### 6.1.2 Breeding stations and distribution of genetic material

The change in China's sheep breeds has been accompanied by a change in the structure of the breeding sector. Liberalization of the sector has also brought about a proliferation in breed service providers.

---

**Box 6.1.** Characteristics of Small Tailed Han sheep.

---

Small Tailed Han sheep have the following traits:

- 2.5 to 3.3 offspring are produced per lambing which occurs three times every 2 years. That is, females produce an average of nine lambs every 2 years.
- Male lambs can reach a liveweight of 35 kg at 5 months of age and 45 kg at 6 months of age but average weights are more like 35 kg at 6 months of age. Feed trial results from one breeding company records that males reach an average of 63 kg at 12 months of age, plus or minus 8 kg over the test flock.
- Mature males grow to an average height (front hoof to shoulder) of 92 cm, and mature females 77 cm.
- Dressing rates bone-in for males are relatively low at around 47% at 6 months of age, and 52% at 12 months of age. Dressing rates bone-out for males are 37% at 6 months of age and 41% at 12 months of age.
- Rams can mate for 4.5 years.
- The sheep were said in Shandong to be adaptable, including to warm, humid areas. Inner Mongolian officials said that they were less hardy than local sheep but grassland regulations entailing a shift from grazing to pen-feeding will increase adaptability.
- The eating quality of lamb or mutton from pure bred Small Tailed Han sheep is generally regarded to be poor.

A breeding company in Inner Mongolia recorded the following birthing rate results from crossing Small Tailed Han sheep ewes with Poll Dorset rams.

- F1 crosses had a similar lambing rate to pure-bred Small Tailed Han sheep (above). In optimal feeding and housing conditions, they believe that the cross can lamb every 8 months and embryo transplants can be done twice per year.
- F2s crossed back to Poll Dorsets lost some of the fecundity, where 65% of the comebacks had one offspring and 35% had multiple births (two to three lambs).
- Results for F3 Poll Dorset comebacks were not available but were expected to be similar to the F2's.

---

The number of registered sheep breeding stations or farms in China rose markedly from 138 in 1996 to 458 in 2003 of which 397 were for meat sheep and 61 for fine wool sheep (Editorial Board of the China Animal Husbandry Yearbook, various years). The most dramatic increase occurred in the central and northern provinces of Shandong, Hebei, Shanxi, Shaanxi, Liaoning and Beijing. In contrast, some of the far northern provinces and autonomous regions of Inner Mongolia, Heilongjiang and Jilin experienced a fall in the number of sheep breeding stations. Over the same period, the total number of breeders in the stations rose from 366,000 to 858,000 in 2003, of which 549,000 were meat breeders and 309,000 were fine wool breeders.[6] The breeding stations sold out a total of 340,000 breeding sheep of which 265,000 were meat sheep.

The rapid increase in the numbers of smaller size breeding stations is a result of liberalization of the sector. At the highest level, a small group of centrally recognized breeding stations were delegated to provincial level. The provincial Animal Husbandry Bureau grants operating licences to all breeding stations which must comply with standards for breeding stock and other criteria. Ownership of former state breeding stations (operating as service units as discussed in Chapter 4) is under transition and corporatization. Many staff of the stations are investing and operating the stations as private or shareholder companies with various bodies within the local government also often holding shares. In addition, new stations are being established. Despite the ownership reforms, the breeding sector remains closely aligned with local government and the Animal Husbandry Bureau in particular. For a detailed budgetary analysis of the economics of sheep breeding farms see Zhang *et al.* (2002).

Traditionally the breeding stations have delivered genetic material – rams, semen and embryos – to grassroots levels in various ways. First, rams can be sold directly to relatively large households (most likely to be in pastoral areas), which run the rams in their flocks for natural mating. The household has to weigh up the benefits of buying their own rams, which can cost several thousand Remimbi, against using the services of the local breed improvement stations or 'ram households' which can charge up to Rmb30 per service.[7] The second sales outlet for breed stations is local (village or township) stations or households which are registered with the local (township or county) Animal Husbandry Bureau and provide breed services on a commercial or semi-commercial basis. In pastoral areas, the rams are often leased out to households to run with their flocks. In agricultural and semi-pastoral areas where the distances are less, households can also take their ewes to the local breed improvement station to be serviced either

---

6. In 2003, 508,000 of the breeding sheep were fertile females and 332,000 of these were meat sheep breeds.
7. Households are charged per successful pregnancy and according to the quality and type of ram. In one semi-pastoral county in Inner Mongolia, the charge was Rmb30 for a mating with a pure Charolais ram. However, the Yuncheng Dapeng Breeding Station in Heze Prefecture in Shandong Province charges only Rmb10 per service of its Small Tailed Han sheep.

through natural mating or artificial insemination. Chifeng City in Inner Mongolia had 500 local level sheep breed improvement points in 2004 and aimed to have 1000 within a few years, many of which would be able to provide breeding services from Poll Dorset, Charolais and Suffolk genetics. The prefecture is seeking 100% artificial insemination coverage for sheep.

Artificial insemination still accounts for a modest part of meat sheep breeding in China, especially when compared to the beef cattle breeding which has a relatively centralized breeding station and artificial insemination station network run by the Animal Husbandry Bureau (see Longworth *et al.*, 2001, Chapter 3). However, China has sought to develop its artificial insemination network for meat sheep breeding in recent years. China has also made large advances in its embryo transfer technology. In 2003, breeding stations produced 17,000 sheep embryos, 15,000 of which were for meat sheep breeds. A further 20,000 sheep and goat embryos were imported between 1998 and 2003. Chifeng City alone has six major breeding centres with the capacity to conduct embryo transfers.

### 6.1.3 Vertical integration in the breeding business

In addition to the traditional though more liberalized sheep breeding structure discussed above, completely new structures have also emerged. Rather than distributing genetic material through the traditional network of lower level breed improvement stations, points and households, many breeding stations or companies have developed closer and more direct or vertically integrated relationships with producers.

In Heze Prefecture in Shandong Province for instance, breeding companies often 'loan' linked households a Small Tailed Han breeding ewe which is then crossed with a ram held by the breeding company. The household returns replacement females to the company or to other households in the programme. The males are retained by the household to feed and sell. Because of the high productivity of the Small Tailed Han sheep (of around nine lambs every 2 years), however, the household also has opportunity to keep females to expand the household flock. Both the breeding farm and the household therefore expand sheep numbers to build up flocks or for sale. This arrangement minimizes feeding, shedding and other costs for the breeding company, and provides households the opportunity to scale up their operations without significant cash outlay.

Numerous examples of this type of relationship occur in Heze and reflect developments in other parts of China and for other livestock types. One breeding company in Liangshan County of Heze Prefecture (the Liangyang Breeding Sheep Farm) had informal relationships with about 1000 households. The Yuncheng Dapeng Breeding Station – which used to be a county level Animal Husbandry Bureau breeding station but has now been bought out by former Animal Husbandry Bureau officials to become a shareholder company – keeps most of its sheep with linked households and sells between 40,000 and 50,000 head outside of the county every year.[8]

Some of these arrangements are also tied in with poverty alleviation programmes in Heze Prefecture. As overviewed in Chapter 5, the Shan County Sheep Breeding Station had distributed about 4000 sheep to poverty stricken households in 2003 as part of a joint breed improvement and poverty alleviation programme. It had bred up numbers in the station to 7000 head and was aiming for 13,500 head by 2005.

In addition, links between breeding companies and households are strengthened through networks and associations. For example, Liangshan County has a Small Tailed Han sheep association comprised of 40 to 50 members in 14 townships in the county. Each household raises about 200 head to total 150,000 head or 30% of the flock in Liangshan County. Many households have entered into the potentially lucrative breeding sheep market where breeding sheep can be worth several thousand yuan rather than several hundred yuan as slaughter sheep. These breeding companies and households are integrated into the breeding market – including households in other regions looking to raise Small Tailed Han sheep – through a loose network of speculative traders, markets, associations and livestock officials.

**Box 6.2.** Profile of the Lukang company.

The Lukang company was established in 1997 in Wongniute County, Chifeng City in Inner Mongolia. It is a private company engaged in sheep breeding but with plans to integrate into downstream activities. The company itself held 3000 breeding sheep in four facilities in 2004 with a total capacity of 4000 head. Each of these facilities consists of hundreds of mu of shedding (with a construction cost Rmb100 per square metre) and land for crop and fodder production. The main breeds are Small Tailed Han sheep ewes crossed with Poll Dorset, Charolais, Suffolk and Merino rams. The company does some artificial insemination and embryo transplant work which will be given more emphasis in the future. Feed for the rams consisted of 1 to 1.25 kg of fodder per day (of this, straw makes up 80% and lucerne 20%) with an additional 0.5 kg of concentrate feed (soybean meal, maize and sunflower cake). The daily weight gain for the crosses is around 200 g. In 2004 the company had sold breeding sheep in northern China (Liaoning and Heilongjiang) through Animal Husbandry Bureau contacts and networks.

In addition to the breeding sheep business, Lukang has also integrated in the slaughter sheep business. It has sold 20,000 sheep at a cost of Rmb300 each to 2000 households. The capital (Rmb6 million) is loaned to the households through the local agricultural cooperative while various local government bodies pay the interest payments for the households. The company markets their sheep or buys them back. Some males have been sold by the company for slaughter to Beijing (Jinxiu Dadi Company) and Chengde in Hebei Province (Fashun Company) for Rmb7 per kg liveweight. The increased number of slaughter sheep available in the future will be sold direct to abattoirs or on local markets. In 2004 the company was looking for partners and capital to integrate from sheep breeding and production into these trading and slaughter activities.

---

8. Yuncheng County sells out 100,000 to 150,000 head to large households, many of which have also registered as individual companies. One such example is the Dingtao Lubao small tail sheep farm with about 600 head.

These companies and households are highly exposed to the notoriously volatile breeding market where the value of breeding livestock can drop very dramatically.[9] This risk is particularly high for Small Tailed Han sheep because of the large numbers produced and the limitations of the breed mentioned above. As an indication of this, the profits from the production and sale of Small Tailed Han ewes from Heze fell from Rmb1500 in 2002 to Rmb800 in 2003, although this was partly blamed on the transport restrictions imposed by the SARS outbreak.

Another fieldwork site not dominated by Small Tailed Han breeds – Chifeng City in Inner Mongolia – also has many breeding companies integrated with households. For example, the Santai Sheep Company in Ningcheng County (see Box 6.3 and Image 6.1) was established in 2002 by two private investors (with 50% of the shares) and the Ningcheng County Poverty Alleviation Office (with the other 50%). The poverty alleviation office provides an interest free loan to the local households to buy the breeding sheep (at about Rmb10,000 per head for a Poll Dorset ram) which is then paid back over time.

A major privately owned company called Lukang in Wongniute County runs a 'core flock' of 3000 breeding sheep (see Box 6.2). Lukang plans to distribute 20,000 sheep to households within the county and to become the biggest sheep company in Inner Mongolia. A loan facility of Rmb6 million from an Agricultural Credit Cooperative will provide households a loan of Rmb300 to buy the sheep with the county government paying the interest on the loans. The company already conducts embryo transfers and will move toward 100% artificial insemination coverage. Lukang has built a live sheep market, and plans to build an abattoir.

In another example, the Songshan Embryo Transplant Centre in Chifeng City established a meat sheep association with 10,000 household members from

**Box 6.3.** Profile of the Santai company.

The Santai company was established in December 2002 and is based in Ningcheng County, Chifeng City in Inner Mongolia. The shareholder company is 50% owned by two private investors and 50% owned by the Lingcheng County Poverty Alleviation Office. In 2004, the central breeding farm had imported 300 Poll Dorsets (both male and female) and held several hundred Small Tailed Han ewes. The male offspring are sold to breeding households at township level for up to Rmb10,000 per head. The females are sold for Rmb400 per head to households that belong to small sheep raising areas in the natural village.[10] Santai has links with three of these small areas in the natural village, which also form an association. Each small area consists of about 20 sheep raising households that hold 20 to 30 sheep each. That is, about 1500 ewes bred by Santai are raised in local households.

---

9. For example, in the neighbouring prefecture to Heze – Zhoukou Prefecture in Henan Province – one household interviewed bought 3 Boer breeding goats for Rmb40,000 each from the Henan Animal Husbandry Bureau in 2002 which were worth only Rmb4000 each by 2004. He likened the breeding sector to a casino. There are more recent parallels for household purchases of imported dairy cattle.
10. A natural village (*ziran cun*) is the lowest and an informal level of organization equivalent to a work team in pre-reform China.

**Box 6.4.** Profile of the Hongwu company.

The Hongwu Group based in Chifeng City in Inner Mongolia is a private company with a registered capital of Rmb237million. It is involved in a diverse range of business activities including mining, distilling and frozen food. The company established a cattle feedlot in 1993 that now has a 500 head capacity and also has an abattoir that has a capacity to slaughter 100 cattle and several hundred sheep per day, although it operates for only 3 months of the year in summer. Hongwu also took over a dairy operation in 2001 but it was closed by 2004. The food activities of the company are also integrated with a small chain of Hongwu hot pot restaurants.

The Hongwu Group is recognized as an Inner Mongolia-level vertically integrated dragon head enterprise in the livestock industry. As such, it has been provided with special funding, part of which was used to start the meat sheep breeding and services operation in 2000. The initial investment from the company itself was Rmb6 million in sheds, Rmb7 million in sheep and additional working capital. The company was also provided with land by the local (Hongshan district) government and was exempt from fees and taxes in initial years of establishment.

The breeding centre is located on the outskirts of Chifeng City and consists of 2000 mu of land, about 500 mu of forage and 132 large brick sheds to house sheep. The breeding programme is based around crossing introduced rams (including Dorset, Suffolk, Charolais and German Merino) with Small Tailed Han ewes. Company officials claimed that the F1 offspring of these crosses can weigh 40 kg at 6 months old if fed well. They are not suited to grazing for more than a couple of (warm) months per year but are better suited than local breed sheep for shed feeding. The reported 55% dressing percentage of the F1 sheep is much higher than the local sheep of 35%, while the meat yield from carcass of the F1s was reported at 80%. The company was also seeking to develop its own Hongwu breed.

The breeding centre housed 12,000 sheep in 2002, 7000 sheep in 2003 but very few when revisited in 2005. The numbers of sheep sold or distributed also fell. In 2002 the company sold 3000 breeding ewes (for Rmb800 to Rmb900 throughout Inner Mongolia, Liaoning and Hebei), 2000 lambs (20 kg liveweight at 6 months old for Rmb350) and slaughtered 1000 lambs themselves (and claimed to sell the boned-out meat for Rmb36 per kg). The company also provided breeding services (at a rate of Rmb30 per successful pregnancy).

By 2005, sales had decreased significantly and were conducted through direct links with households. By 2005 Hongwu had sold (at a price of Rmb800) a total of 4000 ewes to households in four production bases in various parts of Inner Mongolia. Households raise the sheep based on breeding, feeding and veterinary regimes set by Hongwu. Indeed, the semen straws come from Hongwu while the artificial insemination is done by local Animal Husbandry Bureau stations. The company then buys back the lambs when they reach at least 8 months or 40 kg liveweight. Purchase prices in 2004 were Rmb7 to Rmb7.4 per kg liveweight. The sheep are purchased in August during the busy slaughter season. If profitable, Hongwu can then feed the lambs in the company feedlot for another month before slaughter.

The company originally had plans to turn off 100,000 sheep per year and to extend the model to cattle production. The plans, however, have been abandoned. It appears that after the initial years of subsidized establishment, the high costs of the breeding operation were unable to be recouped given the prevailing prices for breeding sheep and lambs.

20 nearby townships. The households have to pay service and association fees to the breeding centre. In exchange the breeding centre provides breeding services and can also market the sheep and lamb for the households in bigger lots.

Other more widely known examples of breeding centres selling breeding sheep to households are overviewed for the Hongwu Group in Box 6.4 and the Kangda Group in Box 6.5. Reflecting the dynamic and risky nature of the industry, the breeding activities and their links with households have been wound back substantially and had stopped or stalled by 2005.

The vertically integrated 'breeding company + household' model is closely related to other production aspects of the industry discussed below, including the organization of households by local government and the provision of services by the Animal Husbandry Bureau such as the construction of sheep pens and the

---

**Box 6.5.** Profile of the Kangda company.

---

The ambitious plans of Kangda to become the largest company in the Chinese sheep industry are outlined below based on a visit to the company in Daxing District in the outskirts of Beijing in 2003 and on articles by Kangda Group (2002) and Kangda Group (2003). However, follow-up questioning and a revisit in 2005 revealed that the plans had not come to fruition and indeed that the company was barely operating.

The most tangible outcome of the plans was the construction of a sheep breeding centre that still exists today, albeit drastically scaled down. In 2003, thousands of breeding sheep were held in temperature controlled and television monitored rooms. Breeds included Charolais, Romani, German Merinos and Boer goats. The website (www.sinosheep.com) was operating between 2002 and 2004 and contained an enormous amount of information on the Chinese sheep industry and provided a forum for business activities.

Like many other breeding companies in China, the breeding operations were to be linked to downstream sectors. The Kangda Company and the Daxing Animal Husbandary Bureau established the Daxing Meat Sheep Association which was to involve 10,000 households in 50 small specialized sheep raising areas with a total flock 350,000 meat sheep and a turnoff of 600,000 head. Many townships in Daxing were to contain several small areas which were to be merged with other nearby townships to form a 'small association' that was to feed into the larger Daxing association. The network of small areas, townships and associations were to be organized around the Kangda Company, which would contract directly with the households.

Daxing is poor relative to urban areas in Beijing and is also a Hui minority area. Thus significant government funding – Rmb27 million for buildings alone – was made available for the project. The households were also to invest in sheep and buildings (up to Rmb200,000 each) where the Beijing Animal Husbandry Office undertook to provide services and help them with loans while Kangda undertook to act as a guarantor for the loans. Despite these plans and resourcing efforts, by 2005 the scheme had been abandoned.

The other major part of the Kangda plan was to build the largest sheep abattoir in Asia with a capacity 4000 head per day on an 8 h shift. The walls of the abattoir had been constructed in 2003 but stalled soon after because bank loans for the project had been withdrawn. However, the designated slaughter point located next to the proposed abattoir area was slaughtering, butchering and distributing sheep meat.

---

development of feed and grazing systems. The Central government through the Animal Husbandry Bureau provides Rmb5 million and Inner Mongolian government provides Rmb30 million per year for breeding activities. This is eclipsed by local-level funding for various production subsidies, credit subsidies and poverty alleviation programmes. Thus the breeding sector is becoming corporatized in so far as the sector is privatizing, but still within the context of government guidance, participation and investment.

The sector is also beginning to resemble state farm systems where 'core flocks' are tightly controlled by a central organization and households fit into their programme in the areas of breed extension and sheep production. The reversion to centrally based systems reflects the market failures that can arise with livestock breeding, especially with small scale and fragmented industry structures.

## 6.2 Sheep production

China's sheep production sector is highly heterogeneous and in a state of flux due to the growth of the industry and developments in sectors such as breeding. Some insights into household sheep production in various areas and years were provided in the budget analysis in Chapter 3. The discussion below provides a snapshot of the structure of the sector in 2002 based on the scale of production data presented in Table 6.1.

Like most livestock industries in China, the sheep and goat industries have a low scale of production. Households like those shown in Image 6.2 that turn off one to 49 sheep or goats per year account for about 74% of total turnoff in the industry. With some exceptions, the production and marketing systems for these small households is very fragmented. Livestock are raised by households that operate on an individual basis and sold to private dealers, and are destined for low value markets.

Of more interest to agribusiness concerns are the specialized producers that turn off more than 50 head of sheep or goats per year and have the capacity to target higher value market segments.[11] These include large scale households and medium sized households that are able to cooperate with other similar households and are well integrated into the industries, as well as state farms.

---

11. There is no formal definition of a specialized sheep or goat raising household in China. As a rule of thumb, if 60% of a household's income is generated from a particular activity, then it can be deemed to be specialized in that activity. However, it is more common to define specialization in terms of absolute numbers in stock. Various government officials and academics stated that a sheep raising specialized household holds: more than 50 adult sheep in agricultural areas; more than 100 adult sheep in semi-pastoral areas; and more than 150 adult sheep in a pastoral area. However, definitions of a specialized household vary enormously by region. For example, some agricultural areas visited in Shandong regarded a household as specialized in sheep and goat production if it holds more than five head. In some pastoral and semi-pastoral areas such as Chifeng Prefecture in Inner Mongolia, the cut-off point is set as high as 200 head of stock.

**Table 6.1.** Scale of sheep and goat production in China and by province, 2002.

| | 1–4 head | | | 5–49 head | | | 50–199 head | | | 200–499 head | | | 500–999 head | | | Over 1000 head | | |
|---|---|---|---|---|---|---|---|---|---|---|---|---|---|---|---|---|---|---|
| | Producers | Turnoff* | % | Producers | Turnoff* | % | Producers | Turnoff* | % | Producers | Turnoff* | % | Producers | Turnoff* | % | Producers | Turnoff* | % |
| All China | 31,449,222 | 84,051,000 | 33 | 6,174,746 | 10,451,920 | 41 | 546,951 | 4,937,280 | 19 | 45,084 | 1,311,990 | 5 | 6,596 | 426,900 | 2 | 1,518 | 253,140 | 1 |
| Beijing | 8,311 | 26 | 1 | 30,078 | 71,990 | 27 | 8,757 | 89,980 | 34 | 1,080 | 33,260 | 13 | 444 | 30,750 | 12 | 141 | 35,260 | 13 |
| Tianjin | 210 | 1 | 0 | 4,293 | 12,500 | 69 | 256 | 3,850 | 21 | 50 | 1,560 | 9 | 1 | 60 | 0 | 0 | 0 | 0 |
| Hebei | 2,049,709 | 5,972 | 35 | 458,564 | 1,087,150 | 46 | 71,857 | 586,500 | 25 | 2,186 | 76,410 | 3 | 275 | 20,080 | 1 | 19 | 3,660 | 0 |
| Shanxi | 535,103 | 1,799 | 30 | 100,671 | 221,550 | 37 | 19,993 | 163,870 | 27 | 892 | 26,220 | 4 | 73 | 4,480 | 1 | 30 | 3,220 | 1 |
| Inner Mongolia | 676,806 | 2,075 | 10 | 494,421 | 690,590 | 34 | 72,217 | 561,710 | 28 | 10,343 | 307,030 | 15 | 2,851 | 175,030 | 9 | 819 | 98,070 | 5 |
| Liaoning | 175,647 | 369 | 11 | 79,218 | 156,700 | 49 | 16,142 | 102,250 | 32 | 888 | 21,630 | 7 | 37 | 2,120 | 1 | 10 | 1,100 | 0 |
| Jilin | 186,536 | 445 | 16 | 41,815 | 99,570 | 35 | 16,514 | 121,790 | 43 | 448 | 13,180 | 5 | 69 | 4,860 | 1 | 3 | 950 | 0 |
| Heilongjiang | 56,506 | 177 | 6 | 37,736 | 110,940 | 35 | 10,306 | 113,240 | 35 | 2,001 | 63,010 | 20 | 193 | 11,210 | 4 | 22 | 3,720 | 1 |
| Shanghai | 0 | 0 | 0 | 16,146 | 42,800 | 84 | 613 | 5,340 | 11 | 6 | 170 | 0 | 2 | 150 | 0 | 13 | 2,370 | 5 |
| Jiangsu | 3,213,953 | 8,710 | 47 | 534,514 | 757,860 | 41 | 15,369 | 170,420 | 9 | 1,372 | 40,950 | 2 | 37 | 2,540 | 0 | 10 | 2,650 | 0 |
| Zhejiang | 503,236 | 1,243 | 69 | 14,007 | 32,350 | 18 | 2,488 | 21,950 | 12 | 49 | 2,240 | 1 | 6 | 360 | 0 | 0 | 0 | 0 |
| Anhui | 2,589,318 | 4,955 | 44 | 531,877 | 477,330 | 42 | 11,276 | 142,270 | 13 | 403 | 13,770 | 1 | 16 | 930 | 0 | 3 | 400 | 0 |
| Fujian | 123,507 | 304 | 29 | 19,155 | 42,840 | 41 | 2,674 | 24,490 | 24 | 169 | 5,390 | 5 | 9 | 600 | 1 | 0 | 0 | 0 |
| Jiangxi | 222,063 | 512 | 51 | 34,395 | 27,830 | 28 | 3,351 | 19,500 | 19 | 63 | 1,520 | 2 | 5 | 320 | 0 | 0 | 0 | 0 |
| Shandong | 4,515,776 | 13,623 | 35 | 714,643 | 1,711,230 | 44 | 65,917 | 724,570 | 19 | 3,079 | 100,270 | 3 | 130 | 9,940 | 1 | 20 | 5,400 | 0 |
| Henan | 5,864,130 | 17,366 | 48 | 971,784 | 1,469,400 | 41 | 36,888 | 345,520 | 10 | 1,649 | 52,090 | 1 | 125 | 8,460 | 0 | 17 | 3,490 | 0 |
| Hubei | 444,511 | 905 | 32 | 68,993 | 121,160 | 43 | 7,303 | 60,240 | 21 | 343 | 10,320 | 4 | 10 | 660 | 0 | 1 | 170 | 0 |
| Hunan | 999,295 | 2,482 | 31 | 132,366 | 380,130 | 47 | 21,355 | 143,780 | 18 | 1,077 | 30,660 | 4 | 76 | 4,320 | 1 | 3 | 520 | 0 |
| Guangdong | 13,310 | 31 | 11 | 4,195 | 12,720 | 46 | 771 | 8,540 | 31 | 40 | 1,500 | 5 | 20 | 1,320 | 5 | 4 | 620 | 2 |
| Guangxi | 556,992 | 965 | 54 | 29,948 | 65,090 | 36 | 1,606 | 13,270 | 7 | 135 | 3,760 | 2 | 10 | 980 | 1 | 0 | 0 | 2 |
| Hainan | 400,534 | 773 | 86 | 11,555 | 12,600 | 14 | 13 | 80 | 0 | 1 | 20 | 1 | 1 | 50 | 0 | 0 | 0 | 0 |
| Chongqing | 595,898 | 1,568 | 56 | 98,750 | 93,580 | 34 | 2,906 | 22,930 | 8 | 130 | 3,260 | 1 | 13 | 970 | 0 | 0 | 0 | 0 |
| Sichuan | 3,783,226 | 8,899 | 57 | 446,866 | 547,240 | 35 | 10,686 | 84,990 | 5 | 1,125 | 25,040 | 2 | 52 | 3,450 | 0 | 7 | 1,960 | 0 |
| Guizhou | 453,682 | 1,213 | 42 | 123,311 | 125,570 | 43 | 4,853 | 39,370 | 14 | 100 | 3,010 | 1 | 10 | 610 | 0 | 1 | 110 | 0 |
| Yunnan | 855,119 | 1,838 | 46 | 107,841 | 152,990 | 38 | 5,280 | 49,220 | 12 | 128 | 4,530 | 1 | 100 | 7,340 | 2 | 10 | 1,780 | 1 |
| Xizang | 54,057 | 209 | 4 | 148,607 | 481,810 | 89 | 2,574 | 38,610 | 7 | 0 | 0 | 0 | 0 | 0 | 0 | 0 | 0 | 0 |
| Shaanxi | 786,338 | 1,888 | 43 | 194,995 | 158,890 | 36 | 14,027 | 86,440 | 20 | 256 | 6,030 | 1 | 15 | 900 | 0 | 5 | 610 | 0 |
| Gansu | 725,813 | 2,810 | 48 | 139,808 | 214,340 | 37 | 9,765 | 74,010 | 13 | 285 | 7,020 | 1 | 7 | 460 | 0 | 62 | 8,200 | 1 |
| Qinghai | 130,181 | 462 | 9 | 73,794 | 136,550 | 27 | 24,320 | 202,120 | 40 | 3,812 | 93,090 | 18 | 422 | 25,670 | 5 | 12 | 1,350 | 0 |
| Ningxia | 286,213 | 525 | 18 | 142,059 | 95,910 | 34 | 13,454 | 94,640 | 33 | 1,317 | 30,850 | 11 | 122 | 6,890 | 2 | 16 | 3,650 | 1 |
| Xinjiang | 643,242 | 1,907 | 8 | 368,341 | 840,710 | 36 | 73,420 | 821,790 | 35 | 11,657 | 334,200 | 14 | 1,465 | 101,390 | 4 | 290 | 73,880 | 3 |

*Indicates turnoff per year.

*Source:* Ministry of Agriculture, unpublished.

### 6.2.1 *Scale of sheep and goat production*

Scale of production data provides some useful insights into the heterogeneity of the production sector of livestock industries in China. In particular, larger scale producers tend to have higher technical capabilities and target higher value markets, while the converse is true of smaller scale producers. Table 6.1 provides national and provincial level data for 2002 on scale of sheep and goat production. Figure 6.1 highlights some of this scale of production information for China as a whole as well as for the key pastoral region of Inner Mongolia and the key Central Plains agricultural province of Shandong.

This scale of production data contains several serious limitations. First, the data do not differentiate between sheep and goats, or meat sheep and fine wool sheep. Second, data previous to 2002 are not publicly available, while more recent data available in the *China Animal Husbandry Yearbook* (2004) aggregate many of the scale categories, precluding comparisons across years. Third, the data refer to sheep and goat turnoff, rather than 'in stock' which is the basis used to define specialization in China. The relationship between numbers in stock and turnoff is highly variable depending on breed, production system, region and type (or scale) of producers.

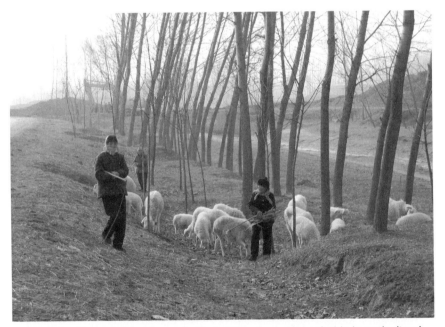

**Image 6.2.** Sheep-raising households in Shandong. Households in agricultural areas combine their few head of sheep to graze along the road while collecting firewood. Small scale households dominate the sheep production sector. Women and children are often responsible for husbandry work.

The 2002 data shows that for China as a whole, one-third of all sheep and goats are turnedoff by households that turnoff one to four sheep or goats per year, two-fifths by households that turnoff between five and 49 head, and one-fifth by households that turnoff 50 to 199 head. Around 8% of sheep and goats are turnedoff by producers that turnoff more than 200 head.

Figure 6.1 reveals that scale of production is larger in pastoral regions such as Inner Mongolia compared with agricultural areas such as Shandong. Fieldwork observations suggest, however, that the scale of production is increasing in Shandong. With respect to regions not shown in Figure 6.1, one third of the sheep turnedoff in Beijing come from farms that turnoff in excess of 200 head with 13% on farms with a turnoff in excess of 1000 head. In many of the provinces in southeastern China, where there is a high proportion of goats, most goats are turnedoff by households that turn off between one and four head. The scale of production is also low in many of the southwestern provinces (including Sichuan, Guizhou, Guangxi and Chongqing).

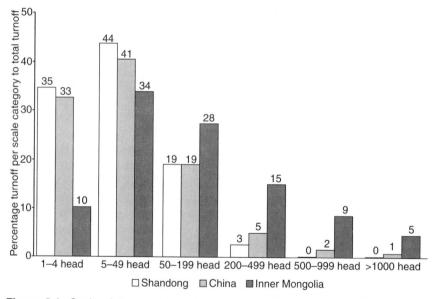

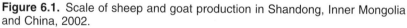

**Figure 6.1.** Scale of sheep and goat production in Shandong, Inner Mongolia and China, 2002.

The scale of production for sheep and goat production is relatively large compared to other livestock industries. While significant proportions of sheep and goats are self consumed by households in China, the vast majority are raised for feeding and sale outside the household system. This contrasts with the multitude of 'one cow households' that raise cattle for draught and transport purposes and households that feed a few pigs or a few chickens on family scraps.

### 6.2.2 Large scale producers

For the purposes of discussion, large scale producers in the Chinese context are defined as having an annual turnoff in excess of 200 head. In 2002 the annual turnoff from producers with a turnoff of more than 200 head was 19.92 million head, which accounts for 8.5% of all sheep and goat turned off in China (232.8 million head). This figure is small given that an annual turnoff of 200 head is a generous definition of a large producer, in that the figure includes breeding and state farms.

Table 6.1 shows that Inner Mongolia and Xinjiang accounted for more than 50% of large scale producers. Most of the producers fell in the 200 to 499 head per year turnoff range. Producers in the 500 to 999 range accounted for 12% of large scale producer numbers and 21% of total turnoff from these producers. Only 1518 producers turned off in excess of 1000 head. These very large scale producers are located mainly in the pastoral provinces of Xinjiang, Inner Mongolia and Gansu. However, by 2003 Central Plains agricultural provinces such as Shandong, Beijing, Henan and the northeastern provinces of Liaoning, Jilin and Heilongjiang each had significant numbers (dozens) of producers that turned off more than 1000 head per year (Editorial Board of the China Animal Husbandry Yearbook, 2004).

Two types of producers turn off more than 200 head per year and therefore fall into the large scale category. First, some households in pastoral areas of China run large flocks of sheep in extensive grazing systems. However, even the major pastoral regions of Inner Mongolia and Xinjiang each had a maximum of 13,000 such households in 2002.[12] This small number is significant given that much of the higher value sheep meat in China comes from these provinces, and suggests that many of these sheep are sourced from medium sized producers discussed in the next section.

Several households that turnoff more than 200 head per year were visited on fieldwork. In eastern Inner Mongolia large households often ran 200 to 300 breeding ewes which were local breed Merino crosses in semi-pastoral systems. In the highland pastoral areas of Gansu, sheep tended to be local sheep or improved with Alpine Merinos (see Image 6.3). In all cases, large pastoral households run the sheep in mixed grazing with goats and cattle and/or yaks. To run such large numbers of livestock, households need to be able to access large parcels of land, either through favourable land allocation or by leasing land from other households. Land area grazed and livestock numbers are notionally balanced by administratively set stocking rates. However, the greatest constraint on livestock numbers is the amount of cropping, forage and cutting land available. Households have to feed livestock intensively over winter when pastures are under snow. In addition, new grassland regulations being implemented throughout most of the pastoral

---

12. Numbers in Inner Mongolia do not appear to have increased significantly, but by 2003 there were more than 40,000 households in Xinjiang that turned off more than 100 head per year.

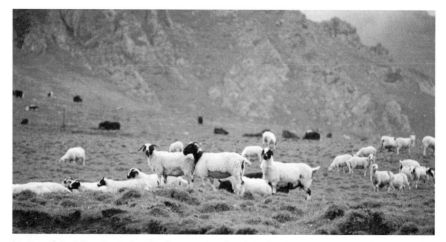

**Image 6.3.** Mixed grazing in Gansu. A mixed flock of goats, sheep and yaks are grazed in highland summer pastures in Gansu.

region have extended the period – sometimes to the whole year – that livestock have to be penned and fed intensively (see Section 5.2.2). The intensification of systems requires a significant increase in investment in sheep housing, pasture, cropping, fencing and water. These costs are only partly offset by various project subsidies which tend to be more available to larger households.

In normal years not subject to severe drought or snow, the ewes have pregnancy, lambing and survival rates of above 90% each. Most ewes in Inner Mongolia are joined in autumn when the ewes and grasslands are in the best condition, and produce 'winter lambs' which are weaned by late spring. Some households will seek to become even larger by keeping replacement lambs, while others will sell slaughter lambs without putting pressure on the grasslands at critical periods of recovery and growth in late spring and early summer. Because of the better technical and management capabilities of large households, they are most likely to integrate into higher value marketing channels that require lambs as young as 6 months old. However, even large households often sell older (up to 3 year old) sheep to local traders for slaughter in local slaughter points.

---

13. Attempts were not made to comprehensively investigate the economics or productivity of the sheep feedlots visited on fieldwork. Feed trial results for Chinese Merinos in Inner Mongolia are reported in China Sheep Association (no date-a), while feed trials and carcass test results for Han crosses with Romney and Polled Dorsets are reported in Zhao (1998, 1999). At the Lukang and Santai breeding companies, Small Tailed Han sheep crossed with various introduced breeds (Poll Dorset and Charolais) reached about 20 kg liveweight at 60 days of age (weaning), and 40 to 50 kg a at 180 days (slaughter age), with a 48% dressing percentage (bone in). For roughage, the sheep were fed 1 to 1.25 kg of maize straw (80%) and lucerne (20%) per day at a total cost for Rmb0.2 per day. For concentrate, the sheep were fed an additional 0.5 kg of soybean meal, maize and sunflower cake at a cost of Rmb0.7 per day. Daily weight gain was said to be between 220 and 270 g per day.

A second form of large scale sheep producers is feedlots, numbers of which appear to have increased in recent years. Of the 53,000 producers that turned off more than 200 head of sheep and goats in China in 2002, more than half of these were in agricultural provinces, with many of the remainder located in agricultural or semi-pastoral parts of pastoral provinces. Although some of these are breeding stations, most are large intensive feeding households or fully fledged feedlots. Unlike the large pastoral households discussed above, these feedlots purchase in most of their lambs and feed them intensively to slaughter age.[13]

A large feedlot of 10,000 sheep owned by the Production and Construction Corps Regiment 129 (Division 7) farm was visited near Kuitun in Xinjiang (see Image 6.4). In addition to acting as a feedlot, the facility is developing a new meat Merino breed of sheep that is a cross of Romney rams and the Production and Construction Corps type Chinese Merinos. These sheep are fed on silage and crushed maize produced by the feedlot company. Labourers working in the feedlot are paid according to the number of sheep they look after per day (at a rate of Rmb0.04 per head per day) and must compensate the feedlot if death rates exceed 6% of the sheep they are responsible for (even though the veterinary and feed regimes are set by the feedlot). They estimated that lambs can be turned off at a profit of Rmb80 per head after allowing for all costs including depreciation, although this was not verified. The construction cost of the feedlot was Rmb3 million, most of which was provided by the Ministry of Agriculture, while the project is also sponsored by the National Science and Technology Commission. Several interviewees in the area were sceptical about the economic viability of the feedlot and believed that feedlots are showcases for a modern industry. As reported in Han and An (2002) in the case of sheep, and in Longworth *et al.* (2001, Chapter 7) in the case of beef, feedlots in China, as elsewhere, are highly sensitive to feed prices.

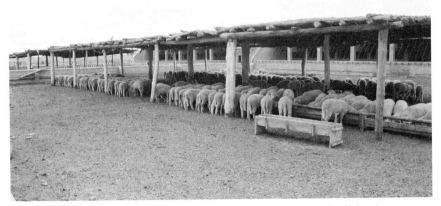

**Image 6.4.** Large feedlot in Xinjiang. Large feedlots are rare in China but there are examples such as that of Regiment 129 (Division 7) Production and Construction Corps farm that breeds and feeds Romney Hill crosses.

### 6.2.3 Mid-sized households and forms of cooperation and specialization

In 2002, China had about 550,000 mid-sized sheep and goat raising households, defined as households that turnoff between 50 and 199 sheep or goats per year. For China as a whole and for Shandong, they accounted for 19% of turnoff while the proportion was higher at 28% in Inner Mongolia.[14] Most of the households in this category produce their own lambs, although there are also small speculative feeding and trading households in agricultural areas of China.

In general, medium sized households do not have the technical capacity or economies of scale exhibited by large households to enter into higher value markets in isolation. However, this capability can be developed by cooperation with other households within specialized sheep producing organizations (see Image 4.1). This cooperation and specialization is not confined to medium sized households, but also encompasses large households and some smaller households.

One form of organization overviewed in Chapters 4 and 5 that has gained currency throughout China is the 'specialized small areas'. Several specialized households (from 5 to 15) combine to create a specialized sheep-producing small area which is based within the confines of the natural village. A natural village (*ziran cun*) is the lowest and an informal level of organization equivalent to a work team in pre-reform China. In Chifeng City alone, there are about 200 specialized sheep and goat-producing small areas that each have at least 1000 head of sheep. In turn, several small areas can combine and cooperate to form a specialized (administrative) village.

One example of a specialized meat sheep small area and village in Chifeng City is in Kalaqin Banner. Some 20 of the 70 households in the village raise sheep. These households each own about 50 Small Tailed Han and Mongolian crosses that were crossed through artificial insemination with Poll Dorsets held by the township sheep breeding station or the household themselves. The village collective provides the land for the area that the sheep were housed and the county Animal Husbandry Bureau provide much of the resources to build the sheds. These are solid sheds with concrete floors, solid fences, and methane converters. Some poverty alleviation money was also contributed. The village Party Secretary acts as the representative of the small area.

Another form of organization involving the participation of specialized households is localized sheep specific associations of which there are many – perhaps hundreds – in China. One example overviewed in Section 6.1 is in Liangshan County in Heze Prefecture where there is a county Small Tailed Han Sheep Association. Branches exist in 14 townships each of which has 40 to 50 specialized household

---

14. Although scale categories differ, in 2003 there were 1.625 million households that turned off between 31 and 100 head of sheep and goats per year, and 159,000 that turned off 100 to 500 head (Editorial Board of the China Animal Husbandry Yearbook, 2004). Gu *et al.* (1998) discuss the resource and market criteria and conditions that should be taken into account in the development of specialized households in Henan.

members. Members of the association raise about 30% of the sheep in the county (500,000), which means that each household holds more than 200 head. Another example, the proposed Daxing Meat Sheep Association, is discussed in Box 6.5.

## 6.2.4 Vertical integration in sheep production and the role of government

Small areas and associations are intertwined with vertically integrated structures in which dragon head enterprises – usually either breeding companies or abattoirs in the sheep meat industry – are also active. In tightly defined relationships, the role of households is confined to the labour of sheep production. The dragon head enterprise dictates feed, breeding and veterinary regimes. Livestock are sold directly to the dragon head, usually at a price slightly higher – Rmb0.1 to Rmb0.2 per kg liveweight higher – than prices on the open market. Although there are examples of such tightly defined relationships, looser arrangements are more common. Under the latter, enterprises provide advice and services to help the household raise sheep to specification, but the household is under no contractual obligation to sell to the enterprise.

Examples of households vertically integrated with breeding companies were discussed above. Some of these examples – including Kangda, Hongwu and Lukang – also had, or planned to develop, abattoir facilities. An example of a relatively loose form of vertical integration between a dedicated slaughter company and sheep meat retailer and sheep producers is the Caoyuan Xingfa Group. In 2004, the company slaughtered about 3 million sheep in abattoirs throughout northwest and northeast China, and bought sheep from about 30,000 households. They had relationships with pastoral households that raise 1 million sheep (more than 10,000 households) in extensive grazing systems, but only bought about 500,000 of these sheep. Households are free to sell to other buyers.

The company claimed that 80% to 90% of the sheep it slaughtered were lambs under 1 year old, known as 'current year sheep', and that it paid Rmb30 or 30% more for these lambs than for mature sheep. Furthermore, the company was trying to encourage households to turn their sheep off at 180 days old, partly to meet the latent demand for this product in the market place, and partly as a means of reducing the seasonality of the slaughter season. This requires relatively well-managed livestock production regimes. Thus the enterprise was working closely with local Animal Husbandry Bureau officials to conduct extension and training programmes and develop new forms of organization. In particular, the aim was to preserve grasslands, minimize livestock mortalities in harsh winters and also meet the specifications of 'dragon head' companies such as Caoyuan Xingfa.

All of the above mentioned forms of organization – small areas, specialized villages, associations and vertically integrated structures – have been developed to overcome the constraints of small scale, household based production and to help dragon head enterprises secure continuity of supply to specification. The government actively encourages these forms of organization. Bodies such as the Animal

Husbandry Bureau provide support in breeding, feeding and veterinary activities and provide a range of support services including training programmes, help in participating in food safety schemes, the construction of sheep housing and the installation of methane converters. From the perspective of government, vertically integrated specialized households are seen as the major vehicle by which livestock industries such as sheep meat can be expanded and commercialized.

Given the large number of households in the industry and the increasingly sophisticated forms of organization to link them with upstream and downstream sectors, it is likely that the specialization and vertical integration models will continue to expand, especially in mid and high value segments of the industry. The longer term outlook of these models depends largely on the development of these higher value markets and the incentives for specialized sheep production households to participate in structures with less government attention and funding. The cases of Hongwu, Kangda and Caoyuan Xingfa overviewed in Boxes 6.4, 6.5 and 7.2 – together with the large number of similar cases in the beef industry (see Longworth *et al.*, 2001) – illustrate the pitfalls of developing large vertically integrated structures.

### 6.2.5 State farms

State farms – including the sheep owned by households living on the state farms – account for a small proportion of China's sheep and goat production. Specifically, in 2002, state farms accounted for only 3.9% of the sheep and goat population, 6.6% of the sheep population, 2.8% of the turnoff of sheep and goats, and 3.7% of the sheep and goat meat output (see Table 6.2).

**Table 6.2.** Sheep and goat production on state farms, 2001 and 2002.

|  | 2001 | | 2002 | |
|---|---|---|---|---|
|  | Quantity | % in China | Quantity | % in China |
| Number of sheep and goats | 11,199 | 3.7 | 12,400 | 3.9 |
| – Of which sheep (1,000 head) | 8,902 | 6.5 | 9,455 | 6.6 |
| Turnoff sheep and goats (1,000 head) | 5,881 | 2.7 | 6,634 | 2.8 |
| Sheep and goat meat (kt) | 103 | 3.5 | 119 | 3.7 |

*Source*: Ministry of Agriculture (2002, 2003a, b).

The vast majority of sheep and goats on state farms are in Xinjiang. State farms in Xinjiang held 8.7 million sheep and goats in 2002, which accounted for 22% of the sheep and goats in the autonomous region, and 70% of all sheep on state farms in China. The high numbers in Xinjiang reflects the importance of the Production and Construction Corps farms which raised 3.9 million sheep in 2002 (see Longworth and Williamson (1993) for a discussion of the Production and Construction Corps systems with regard to sheep production). In other provinces such as Heilongjiang and Hainan where Production and Construction Corp farms operate, state farms also held a significant number of sheep and goats. State farms in Heilongjiang held 870,000 head while those in Hainan held 224,000, accounting for substantial proportions of the sheep and goats in these provinces. State farms in Inner Mongolia raised 1.6 million sheep and goats in 2002, accounting for just 4% of the autonomous region flock.

Despite the relatively low share of production, state farms still exert an influence in the sheep industry for a variety of reasons. State farms have historically been important bases for sheep breeding, especially for fine wool sheep (see Longworth and Williamson, 1993). Many state farms retain a 'core flock' of breeding sheep.[15] However, the vast majority (85% in the case of the Xinjiang Production and Construction Corps system) of the other sheep formerly owned by the state farms have been distributed to households living on the state farms. These households are able to make their own decisions about how to manage and trade their sheep. Like households outside the state farm system, these households are moving out of fine wool production and are increasingly running mixed, local breed, or meat sheep breeds. Some farms however have made a coordinated, farm-led push into meat sheep production which has also involved households on the state farms. Examples include Regiment 129 in Xinjiang (Romney Hills breed) and Jinfeng in Inner Mongolia (Bangde breed). These state farms have become significant producers in higher value markets.

## 6.3 Live sheep marketing

Live sheep are traded through several channels in China. Some involve relatively direct forms of marketing with few intermediaries involved in the trading of breeding sheep or higher value slaughter sheep. However, like other agricultural industries in China, the vast majority of live sheep are traded in low value marketing channels through a network of private dealers and local periodic markets. Many similarities arise with the live cattle marketing system that is discussed in detail in Longworth *et al.* (2001, Chapter 8). However, sheep trading is even more fragmented as sheep are easier to transport and are smaller divisible units of trade. The predominance of specialized larger regional markets is not as evident in sheep marketing as they are for cattle. Nonetheless, significant inter-regional flows of live sheep occur in places such as Inner Mongolia which 'exports' 20% of its live sheep to neighbouring provinces.

### 6.3.1 Direct forms of marketing

Section 6.2 highlighted the relationships between household producers and dragon head enterprises and the incorporation of households into local groups. These production structures are often associated with relatively short supply

---

15. Only a handful of state farms in Xinjiang and Inner Mongolia have maintained fine wool production and breeding activities in recent years. The vast majority of state farms in China are moving out of fine wool or even livestock altogether and into agriculture (especially cotton in Xinjiang) and other industry (Brown *et al.*, 2005).

chains. For example, breeding companies such as Lukang enter into supply arrangements with a limited number of abattoirs (in nearby Beijing and Hebei) to sell not only its own sheep but also those of 2000 households that it is connected with and which are organized into small areas. Other breeding and slaughter companies such as Hongwu and Kangda planned to slaughter sheep that the companies had bred and that were raised by connected households. Slaughter and retail companies such as Caoyuan Xingfa and Xiaofeiyang have flexible arrangements for the purchase of sheep from households. Purchasers for these companies are aware of sheep numbers and types in specific regions and buy directly from the households or through local government, Animal Husbandry Bureau officials, or sometimes local traders and agents.

Relatively direct marketing channels also operate for the trade in breeding sheep. Breeding stations differentiate their sheep by establishing themselves as a company, registering company brands and trademarks, and marketing their sheep outside the rural trade market system. Many of the breeding stations are managed or part owned by former Animal Husbandry Bureau officials who use their knowledge, contacts and networks to market and distribute the sheep. This is particularly effective because the buyers – households, ram households, breeding stations or local government in other production areas – usually also have a close affiliation with the Animal Husbandry Bureau.

### 6.3.2 Markets and dealers

Despite the few direct forms of marketing in China, especially for higher value slaughter and breeding sheep, sheep marketing is dominated by a nexus of household producers, private dealers and slaughter households. Transactions take place mainly on local periodic rural trade markets which serve as a meeting place for direct exchanges to occur between the market participants. There is no systematic or centralized sale of the sheep at the market. All trading is done by direct private treaty. Most of the sheep sold in this way are destined for slaughter in local households or designated slaughter points (see Chapter 7), although some inter-regional traders also operate at these markets.

For an appreciation of how sheep and goats are traded at rural periodic markets, consider the case of the Sunliu Town market in Shan County in Heze Prefecture in Shandong Province. One of 17 markets in the county, it is open every 5 days. It is a large, busy market lining the main road in the town with a large range of produce and commodities. Nevertheless, an area was specifically allocated to sheep and goat trading. Individual farmers took a few head of sheep to the market. Specialized slaughter households and traders then buy the sheep and tie about ten head in the back of a three-wheeled truck (see Image 6.5). Slaughter households purchase in this way every day in various markets and their total purchases and slaughtering numbers are about 3000 per year. There were about ten of this type of truck at the market. The price in December 2003 was about Rmb8 per kg liveweight regardless of whether they were lambs or mature animals.

Households can slaughter both sheep and goats, but because of the predominance of goats in Shan County, most slaughtered goats. Furthermore there was a shortage of sheep in late 2003 and early 2004 because farmers, especially in the North of Heze Prefecture, were trying to build up their flocks as sheep had become more profitable than goats.

Other larger and more specialized markets are located in Miquan on the outskirts of Urumqi in Xinjiang and serve as a major trading point for the whole western area of Xinjiang (Yili, Bole, Tacheng, Altai and Shihezi) to service the urban markets in Urumqi. One of the markets was established as a business operation by the Xinjiang Tianling Animal By-products Company and trades live animals, skins and wool. Around 1.6 million head of livestock were traded in 2002, many of which were winter born lambs which were sold in the May to June period. The other livestock market in Miquan County was owned and managed by the Hualing company which, with a trade of about 1.4 million head of sheep in 2005, was said to be taking business from the Tianling market. Importantly, the Hualing market was linked to a designated slaughter point and meat retail markets also run by Hualing. Like the planned Daxing operation in Beijing (see Box 6.4), Hualing is also building a large modern sheep abattoir.

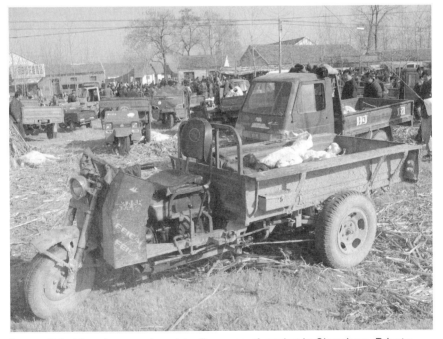

**Image 6.5.** Live sheep and goat trading area of market in Shandong. Private dealers and slaughter households transport sheep and goats in the back of three-wheeled trucks in a market in Heze Prefecture.

Further up the scale of size and specialization is the China Small Tailed Han sheep trading centre in Jiaxiang County in Jining Prefecture in Shandong Province. It is registered as a national level market (hence 'China' in the name of the market). The market was established as a business operation by several private investors with an investment of Rmb16 million and covers an area of 20 ha. Facilities include feed storage, loading and tying facilities while livestock specialists, veterinarians and market personnel are on hand to provide advice, disseminate material and regulations and facilitate and conduct inspections. The market has a holding capacity of 30,000 head of sheep for 600 sellers and has a target of selling 20,000 head per day. In addition, the market can hold 1000 (Luxi breed) cattle and 2000 (Boer breed) goats. The facilities were still under construction in December 2003 but had not formally started trading, so it is difficult to determine the success in filling these ambitions. In addition, a large specialized sheep market was under construction in Wongniute County in Chifeng City in Inner Mongolia. This was closely integrated with the operations of the Lukang company mentioned above.

It is tempting to view the Miquan and Jiaxiang cases as harbingers of future market developments. Yet while markets such as these will continue to emerge (and whither) especially with increasing sophistication and segmentation of the market, small fragmented markets are likely to dominate for some time.

# 7

# Meat sector developments

Having overviewed agribusiness dimensions of live sheep in the previous chapter, this chapter focuses on the flow of sheep meat through the marketing chain. In particular, it examines sheep meat production – sheep slaughter, sheep meat processing, storage and distribution – as well as sheep meat retailing and catering for the domestic trade. As with the live sheep sectors, the sheep meat sector is dominated by highly fragmented and small scale household based operations, but larger, more integrated chains are emerging to target specific market segments. This analysis therefore indicates the way by which agribusiness structures for sheep meat may develop and become more sophisticated.

## 7.1 Sheep meat production

Sheep meat production – incorporating sheep slaughter and sheep meat processing – is conducted by actors that can be classified into three main categories, namely mechanized abattoirs, designated slaughter points and slaughter households. These actors are best considered as existing in a scale continuum, with significant overlap in terms of practices, inputs and outputs. A similar but more detailed classification is also applicable to the cattle slaughter sector as discussed in detail in Longworth *et al.* (2001, Chapter 9). The smaller physical size of sheep, however, means they can be more readily slaughtered by households for their own consumption or for sale, or by restaurants for their own use. Thus the sheep slaughter sector is even more fragmented than the cattle slaughter sector.

The collection of data on slaughter numbers through these channels is problematic. The high level of fragmentation in sheep slaughter precludes local-level officials from collecting accurate sheep slaughter numbers by households, restaurants, or even designated slaughter points. As with other areas of the industry, there is little or no differentiation between sheep and goat slaughter for statistical purposes. Furthermore, although it is certain that only a small proportion of sheep are slaughtered in larger scale, mechanized abattoirs, precise numbers are difficult to collate. Industry officials do not know exactly how many sheep abattoirs there are in China or their capacity, let alone actual throughput. This is partly because of rapid change and ownership transition in the sector and partly because sheep and goat slaughter lines have historically been located in the same plant as cattle abattoirs.

As is the case across all livestock sectors in China, for disease and hygiene reasons, policies are notionally in place to ban the slaughtering of sheep at individual households and for the slaughtering to be done in designated slaughter points or abattoirs. However, the policies have been implemented very unevenly by region and livestock type. In major cities such as Beijing, Xi'an and Hohhot and in smaller cities throughout pastoral regions such as Xinjiang, the policy has been implemented relatively tightly. However, this is not the case in most rural, agricultural areas of China. Although the regulations to move household slaughtering into designated slaughter points has been implemented and enforced relatively tightly for pigs in most regions of China, the same cannot be said for cattle, sheep and goats.

Despite the difficulties in quantifying the structure of the slaughter sector in China, officials in fieldwork regions offered some estimates. In Shandong Province in 2003, sheep slaughtered in abattoirs were estimated to account for only around 15% of the total slaughtered, with the vast bulk killed by slaughter households, either as individuals or in collective designated slaughter points. Less than 1% were killed and consumed by farmers at home for festivals. In Inner Mongolia it was estimated that 10% of the sheep were slaughtered and consumed by farmers at home, 70% by abattoirs and designated slaughter points, and 20% by slaughter households. A profile of the slaughter sector in Beijing appears in Box 7.1.

Cost structures are the major reason for the continued predominance of household slaughtering. A company in Inner Mongolia that slaughters sheep in mechanized abattoirs to produce sheep meat suitable for hot pot dishes indicated a total slaughter cost of around Rmb15 per head. In contrast, slaughter costs for a slaughter household selling into the mass sheep meat market in Beijing or service slaughtering fees for a designated slaughter point will be as low as Rmb1.5 per head. Thus slaughter costs alone place mechanized abattoirs at a competitive disadvantage in selling onto the mass market. Slaughter households do not, however, have the boning, packaging, or cold storage facilities to reach more distant or lucrative markets. Thus the relative importance of the actors in the slaughter sector varies by market segment.

### 7.1.1 *Abattoirs*

The China Meat Association (personal communication, 2004) estimates that there are about 3700 livestock (including poultry) abattoir and meat processing enterprises in China. Of these, 1889 enterprises had annual sales in excess of Rmb5 million in 2004 including 866 abattoirs and 1023 meat processors. Around 25% of these large abattoirs are state owned, with many of the others involving state shareholding.

Of the 3700 enterprises, about 1000 process beef, sheep meat or goat meat, but most are associated only with the slaughter of cattle. Of the sheep and goat operations that do exist, most are linked with cattle abattoirs although as separate slaughter lines. The close relationship between cattle, sheep and goat slaughter in abattoirs is a carry over from the central planning era and the 1980s when the

**Box 7.1.** Major slaughter units and plans in Beijing in 2003.

According to a survey conducted by the Beijing Agricultural Bureau in 2003, there are 64 abattoir and meat processing enterprises in the suburbs of Beijing. These appear to have been defined widely to include small slaughter houses and designated slaughter points. Of these, there were four main sheep slaughter and mutton processing enterprises operating as 'dragon head' enterprises at the city level. The four enterprises were:

- Beijing Kangda Muslim Food Co. Ltd. This company was reported to have an annual slaughter capacity of 560,000 sheep and goats in 2002, with an output of sheep, goat and other processed products of 9750 t. These claims appear to have been exaggerated. In addition, as reported in Box 6.5, the large modern abattoir envisioned by Kangda has not gone ahead and the sheep breeding and production parts of the company have been scaled back or abolished.
- Beijing Fumin Muslim Food Co. Ltd with an annual slaughter capacity of 200,000 sheep and goats in 2002. The company also has a large breeding centre where breeding sheep are raised by households in about 50 villages, and also runs a live animal market.
- Beijing Xiangyun Food Co. Ltd, which had an annual slaughter capacity of 250,000 sheep and goats in 2002.
- Beijing Zhuochen Livestock Co. Ltd, which had an annual slaughter capacity of 200,000 sheep and goats in 2002.

The annual slaughter capacity of the above four 'dragon head' enterprises at city level was 1.21 million sheep and goats in 2002. The turnoff of sheep and goats in Beijing in this year was about 2.64 million. Thus these four enterprises had the capacity to slaughter nearly half of the turnoff of the city. However, estimating the actual numbers or proportions of the enterprises is problematic given the capacities of these enterprises far exceeds actual slaughter numbers, while Beijing imports significant numbers of sheep from outlying provinces. Thus even in a city such as Beijing, slaughter households and designated slaughter points account for the large majority of sheep slaughtered.

According to the Beijing development plan, the municipal government will support ten larger livestock and poultry slaughter and meat processing enterprises, extend their production scale, and improve their product competitiveness at the expense of small slaughter houses and individual butchers.

state built General Food Company abattoirs to meet the needs of Muslim populations in most large cities. As sheep, goat and cattle production has traditionally been associated with pastoralism in China, a significant proportion of counties in the pastoral area have a General Food Company abattoir.[1]

Thus the vast majority of sheep and goat abattoirs in China, as for other livestock abattoirs, were part of the state owned General Food Company network. These General Food Company abattoirs have been subject to reform measures to the point that the vast majority have closed or undergone ownership transition into private or shareholding companies. Excess slaughter capacity within the industry as a whole has hastened the restructuring process. For details on the slaughter plants (*roulianchang*) of the vast General Food Company network, see Waldron *et al.* (2003, Chapter 2).

---

1. Fiscal reforms in the 1980s as well as a concerted effort to increase exports to the Soviet Union also hastened the development of General Food Company abattoirs in pastoral areas. Livestock-based processing activities were viewed as one of the few possibilities for generating revenues for local governments in these areas at the time.

Caoyuan Xingfa was, and perhaps still is, the largest sheep slaughtering company in China. The sheep meat operations of the company were based on the purpose built – albeit antiquated – slaughter lines, cold room facilities, and distribution networks of the General Food Company system. These activities are integrated with food processing, retailing and catering activities. A significant proportion of sheep meat from Caoyuan Xingfa abattoirs enters into the wholesale and rural trade market system, especially lower value and surplus cuts. In 2005, the company managed nationwide marketing and distribution through six large distribution 'districts' and more than 30 offices in provinces throughout China. However, as described in Box 7.2, the company structure and activities changed dramatically in 2006.

In addition to Caoyuan Xingfa, there is a range of other companies that slaughter sheep in China, some of which are listed in Box 7.3. One of the features of the sheep abattoir sector in China is that it is based on rudimentary technology and facilities. Unlike the cattle slaughter sector where there are numerous examples of large modern abattoirs, there were few in the sheep slaughter sector in 2005. The utilization of old, refurbished and in many cases semi-mechanized abattoirs appears to be a cost effective way of meeting the demands of downstream actors in the current market environment. However, as indicated in Box 7.3, many companies are developing or planning a series of new sheep abattoirs, some of which are likely to proceed. As with cattle abattoirs, the viability of these proposed modern abattoirs depends on them securing access to higher value marketing channels (see Longworth *et al.*, 2001, Chapter 9).

Because of the concerted state efforts to facilitate the strategic storage of beef and sheep and goat meat, General Food Companies and their incarnations have access to pre-existing cold storage and delivery systems. For example, the combined cold storage capacity of Caoyuan Xingfa was 35,000 t. Because the slaughter season is highly seasonal in the northern pastoral region, with most slaughtering between August and November, the company must freeze (not chill or vacuum pack) meat for significant periods of time especially as the high consumption season is in winter. The meat is distributed from the cold storage facilities to market or franchised restaurants mostly in distant regions. The company rents (rather than owns) all of the refrigerated trucks required.

Although most sheep meat consumption in China takes place in the immediate area where it was produced, the General Food Company system – together with some new projects[2] and abattoir investments discussed above – mean that substantial inter-regional flows of sheep meat are occurring. For example,

---

2. Some projects have also been established to facilitate sheep meat distribution from remote areas. For instance, the Hong Kong Golden Earl and Ningxia Welfare Industrial Company was reported to have set up a Ningxia–Hong Kong Refrigerator Truck Programme in May 2001. Some 15 cold storage trucks were purchased to ship frozen beef, mutton and other Muslim foods. Four trucks were put into operation to ship more than 300 t of strictly inspected beef, mutton and other agricultural products to Hong Kong (Anon., 2001).

**Box 7.2.** Profile of the Caoyuan Xingfa company.

---

The Inner Mongolia Caoyuan Xingfa began in 1993 as an amalgamation of five township and village enterprises in Yuanbaoshan District of Chifeng City in eastern Inner Mongolia. The company listed on the stock exchange in 1997 and by 2000, the China Meat Association ranked the company in first place of China's sheep meat and yak meat production, third place for chicken meat, and 13th in China's 50 strongest meat enterprises. As late as 2005, the company was recognized as a 'National Leading Agribusiness' by the central government and eligible for a range of preferential policies at national and local levels. The company said that it had 10,000 employees on its books in 2002. However, because of the seasonality of the slaughter season, 6000 of the staff are part time, with around 2500 workers and 1500 technicians employed full time.

The company claimed in interviews in both 2004 and 2005 to have more than 40 abattoirs that slaughter sheep and goats throughout northern China, 20 of which were located in Inner Mongolia. Together, these abattoirs have the capacity to slaughter and process 6 million sheep and goats annually but actual slaughter was said to be closer to 3 million, of which 95% were said to be sheep and only 5% goats. The company had plans to increase slaughter capacity to 10 million sheep. The means and requirements by which Caoyuan Xingfa sourced lambs was discussed in Chapter 6.

Sheep and goat slaughter are just one part of the Caoyuan Xingfa operations. Altogether, the company claimed to own about 60 abattoirs and to lease or have service slaughtering arrangements with a further 40. In addition to sheep and goats, the company slaughters 50 million 'green' chickens annually in six main abattoirs (that have a capacity of 80 million), 200,000 beef cattle, 200,000 yaks in 20 abattoirs in the pastoral region, and various feed facilities. The company had large amounts of unused capacity and aggressive plans to increase throughput. This meat production is combined with other products to produce a bewildering range of thousands of food products, many of which are processed.

On the retailing and catering side, in 2005 the company claimed to have 500 franchised hot pot restaurants, 1000 barbeque restaurants, 1000 Green Food stores and 1000 sections in supermarkets. Autonomous import and export rights were granted in 1997 and around 5000 t of sheep and goat meat was exported including to Japan, the Middle East and Hong Kong. Much of this is goat meat and also cuts for hot pot, skewers, legs, and various Western style cuts. In 2004, the company exported nearly 160,000 live sheep to the Middle East (mainly Jordan), having been restricted in doing so for the previous 8 years because of disease status.

The rise of the Caoyuan Xingfa came to an abrupt end in mid 2006 when the company was declared bankrupt (see Hua and Ke, 2006). The company (including Rmb1.2 billion of its debts) were assumed by the Inner Mongolia Pingzhuang Coal Group, a large state-owned enterprise also based in Yuanbaoshan District. The demise of Caoyuan Xingfa was triggered by questions about its financial accountability and lack of corporate governance. The company can not account for most of the Rmb3 billion that it raised. To hide a series of financial losses, the company over-reported sales revenues in its 2005 (third quarterly) report by more than Rmb330 million. The company raised – but subsequently did not invest effectively or at all – approximately Rmb1 billion for the purpose of buying land and facilities for lamb fattening and feed production (in 2002) and sheep breeding farms, service systems and cooperative arrangements with producer households (in 2003). About half of the 110 'small areas' for green chickens it set up were said to be 'unused'. The company also reported that it received a lower than expected return on the Rmb260 million it invested in 12 food companies (abattoirs) in Inner Mongolia and the company suffered from the outbreak of chicken flu.

---

**Box 7.3.** Other sheep abattoirs in China.

---

Sheep abattoirs other than Caoyuan Xingfa, Hongwu and Kangda (profiled in other boxes) include:

- Sichuan All Star Corporation. This company commenced operation in Ziyang City of Sichuan Province in February 2003. Some US$10 million have been invested to create a Chinese mutton brand to enable Ziyang to export mutton to the international market. It is a key leading enterprise supported by Ziyang City. The total population of slaughtered goats is targeted to reach 4 million by 2005, involving 20,000 farmers with an average of 50 goats per family.

- Gaoyuan Green Food Development Corporation. This company, which is part of the of Qinghai Meat Group, began construction in October 2002 of a large scale beef and mutton processing project with a total investment of Rmb200 million. After completion, it will be a large company involved in beef and sheep slaughtering, processing, product development and distribution.

- The Qinghai Datong Muslim Meat Co. Ltd markets under the brand of 'Lucaoyuan' of beef and sheep meat products. It sells to Beijing and Shanghai as well as northern China. The annual volume of processed products reached 2000 t in 2003 with sales in excess of Rmb30 million.

- The Heze Fushida Food (Food Star) Company. The company has a capacity to slaughter about 2000 sheep and goats per day at its main plant in Yuncheng in Shandong. However, it has another two plants leased from the Wanguang and Yangshan companies. Together the plants have a slaughter capacity of 6000 sheep and goats per day although actual slaughter numbers are much lower at around 600,000 head per annum. The slaughter is predominantly for goats and is unmechanized. Most of the meat is exported (about 5000 t bone-in per year) mainly in frozen full and half carcass pieces for low value markets in the Middle East at around US$1900 per t for lamb meat. The company also has an extensive range of pre-packaged mutton food (especially soup) products.

- Changchun Haoyue Muslim Meat Co. Ltd in Jilin Province. This company slaughtered 150,000 cattle and 50,000 sheep in 2002, and had an annual sales income of Rmb700 million and export value of US$10.5 million.

- As reported in Chapter 6, the sheep production companies of Lukang (Inner Mongolia), Kangda (Beijing) and Hongwu (Inner Mongolia) planned to build purpose-built sheep slaughtering facilities but these had not materialized by 2005.

- Xiaofeiyang has plans to build a substantial slaughter capacity in Inner Mongolia.

- The Hualing abattoir in Urumqi City in Xinjiang had in 2006 nearly completed construction of a modern sheep abattoir using imported equipment. The company claimed that this mechanized plant will more than double its existing 'hand killing' designated point slaughter of 1.4 million head per year.

- Various enterprises are listed on China Feed Web (www.chinafeed.org.cn) that slaughtered more than 10,000 cattle and/or 100,000 sheep or goats in 2002 including Delisi Group (Shandong Province), Henan Bangjie (Henan Province), General Food Company of Shenzhen City (Guangdong Province), Luohe Shuanghui Industry Group (Henan Province) and the General Food Company of Xiantao City (Hubei Province).

---

Inner Mongolia is an important supplier of sheep meat to Beijing and Tianjin as well as neighbouring provinces such as Liaoning, Jilin and Heilongjiang. Indeed various sources claim that Inner Mongolia dominates the supply of mid to high quality sheep meat in China. All major hot pot chains for example claim to source their sheep meat from Inner Mongolia even though cases of false advertising abound.

Another issue important to abattoirs is the degree of butchering and processing at abattoirs. For some markets – especially rural trade and wholesale markets – very little butchering is done at the abattoir. Instead, whole or half carcasses are sent to markets where stallholders butcher according to the needs of the customers. This is especially the case for designated slaughter points and slaughter households discussed below. Abattoirs targeting higher value markets usually have significant boning rooms requiring large numbers of staff. These can produce specific cuts of meat as required by supermarkets for example, to rolls of packaged and frozen sheep meat required for the hot pot trade.

A range of companies have additional facilities to 'deep process' elaborately transformed products. Although sheep meat products do not appear to be subject to the level of transformation of cattle products, there are several examples of enterprises involved in the trade. For example, Baishoufang in Shandong used the products of 200,000 sheep and goats (mainly local goats) to produce products including canned sheep hoof, sheep tripe, sheeps' head meat and sheep soup.

### 7.1.2 Designated slaughter points

Another form of slaughter unit that has become increasingly important in Chinese livestock in recent times is the designated slaughter points. For all livestock types, there are about 50,000 designated slaughter points registered in China, of which 40,000 are county level and below and 10,000 are at the city or prefecture level. Beijing had 67 designated slaughter points in 2004, Shanghai had 52 and Xi'an had 102.

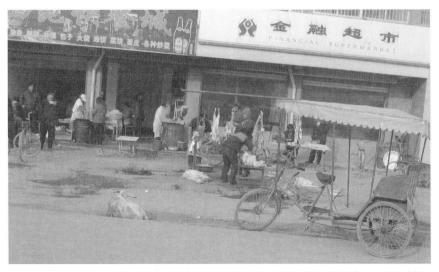

**Image 7.1.** Local-level sheep slaughter and butchering. A butcher in a township in Shandong slaughters sheep on the footpath (in foreground) to sell to passing customers as well as to the restaurant in the background.

Designated slaughter points must register to slaughter specific types of live-stock, and can include mechanized, semi-mechanized or unmechanized facilities. They are often an amalgamation of slaughter households and collectively must reach a set scale in terms of slaughter numbers and people involved. The designated slaughter points and facilities are often collectively operated and can be based on village or township structures.

The designated slaughter points are subject to disease, hygiene and environmental standards, and must pay relevant registration and inspection fees. It is virtually impossible for authorities to police the necessary regulatory standards in an environment dominated by large numbers of small individual slaughter households. Thus designated slaughter points were developed to facilitate conformity to regulations. Although these structures make inspection more feasible, the level of inspection and conditions in the designated slaughter points is highly variable. Designated slaughter points are therefore a product of policy drivers. Nevertheless, there are various marketing and other benefits associated with the collective use of slaughter facilities that has also encouraged their development.

The scale of designated slaughter points – which can slaughter hundreds of sheep per day – facilitates some economies of scale in input sourcing and output marketing. A continuity of supply of sheep can be achieved through local livestock

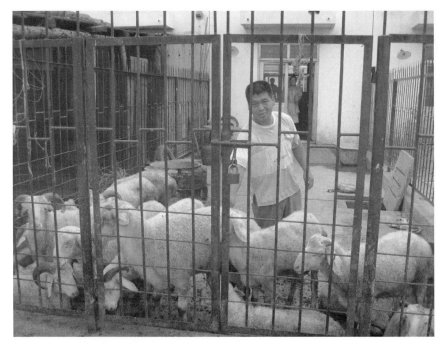

**Image 7.2.** Sheep-holding facilities of a designated slaughter point in a Beijing county. The sheep are held in the pen until ready for slaughter in the slaughter room in the background.

markets or more direct relations with local sheep-producing villages and townships. The continuity of relatively homogeneous product means that slaughter points can service the needs of the lower value end of the hotel, restaurant and institutional trade, or wholesale markets where households from the slaughter point often have stalls. Slaughter points sometimes have their own transport (trucks) and or cold storage facilities. However, outside of winter months, the smaller designated slaughter points – as well as individual slaughter households – have to slaughter in the very early hours of the morning and transport and sell the meat, and especially the offal, within the morning period. Few retail or even wholesale markets have cold storage facilities. It is also significant that the more concentrated structure of designated slaughter points facilitate the collection of by-products such as skins and offal.

Although households that operate at the designated slaughter points utilize common facilities, they usually do so on an individual basis. That is, they butcher and bone the meat in their rooms, employ their own staff, develop their own marketing channels, and often run their own stalls in the markets. Image 7.2 and Image 7.3 provide visual representations of household butchers operating within a designated Muslim slaughter point in Daxing District in Beijing. As mentioned in Section 6.3.2, the Daxing model is similar to that of Hualing in Xinjiang. Indeed, the model of combining an oligopoly designated slaughter point, with live sheep marketing, sheep meat markets, and sometimes mechanized abattoirs

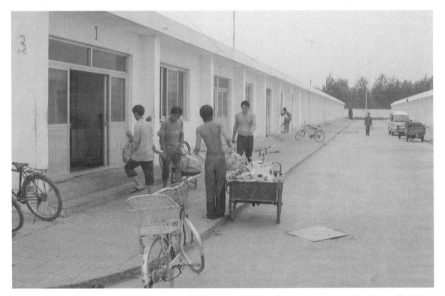

**Image 7.3.** Loading carcasses at a designated slaughter point in Beijing. This is the front of the slaughter room where carcasses are being delivered for further butchering. Note the large number of individual stalls in the collective designated slaughter point.

is becoming more common in some cities in China (such as Beijing, Xi'an and Shanghai) and in both large and small cities in pastoral regions (such as Inner Mongolia and Xinjiang). Designated slaughter points monopolize the slaughter sector of region, prefecture and county level cities/towns throughout Xinjiang.

In most cases, sheep meat from designated slaughter points – as well as from individual households – is butchered prior to being taken to market and usually delivered only rudimentarily in full or half carcasses with the separation of offal. Further butchering is done at the retail or wholesale market outlet according to the needs of the customer.

### 7.1.3 Slaughter households and restaurants

In addition to designated slaughter points, there are a plethora of individual slaughter households that slaughter cattle, sheep and goats although these were not visited on fieldwork. A small slaughter household might kill 10 to 20 sheep and/or goats per day. These households slaughter for local consumption, including households within their village or for local restaurants and stalls. As shown in Image 7.4, local-level distribution occurs through rudimentary means. By-products such as skins are sold to other households and traders specialized in the trade. Image 7.1 shows a butcher in a town in Heze Prefecture with several sheep tied up on the side of the street where he also slaughters and butchers them. The meat from his small stall supplied the small crude restaurant behind him.

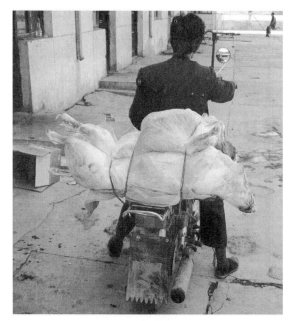

**Image 7.4.** Local-level sheep carcass distribution. Slaughter households delivering meat or restaurants picking up meat often use rudimentary means of transport, such as this motorbike in Gansu.

## 7.2 Sheep meat retailing

Sheep meat markets in China can be categorized into three main groups: retail markets, wholesale markets and supermarkets. As is the case in the slaughter sector, these different retail outlets represent a scale continuum with significant overlap between the categories. For instance, many wholesale markets also conduct retail sales and some large retail markets have company stalls that present products as attractively as many supermarkets. Retail markets dominate the sale of – usually low value – sheep meat in China. However, these and other outlets are evolving to cater for the increasingly sophisticated demands of the food service sector and household consumers.

As background to a discussion about sheep meat retailing and catering, a survey conducted by Wang Jimin and Zhang Cungen from the Institute of Agricultural Economics at the Chinese Academy of Agricultural Sciences in 1998, revealed information about various marketing channels for sheep meat and goat meat in 1998. Wang estimated that retail markets accounted for more than 55% of beef, sheep meat and goat meat sold in China, while supermarkets accounted for only 5%. Around 28% of consumption occurred out of home in restaurants and hotels. Sheep or goats killed and consumed by farmers at home accounted for 6%, with all remaining channels including welfare and gifts accounting for only 5%. Various developments have occurred since the Wang survey in 1998. The proportion of sheep and goat meat sold through retail markets and traded as welfare and gifts has probably declined, while supermarket and out of home consumption has probably increased.

### 7.2.1 Retail markets

There are an enormous number and range of retail markets in China.[3] For example, Shandong has nearly 9000 markets in total, of which about 6600 sell consumer products including food, while 1300 are dedicated food markets (Shandong Statistics Bureau, 2004).[4] Around 94% of consumer products markets are registered at the village level and open periodically. There are 420 dedicated food markets in Shandong that are registered at city level. These are also classed as retail markets but are larger, more sophisticated and offer a wider range of products than do the lower level retail markets.

Beijing has approximately 36,400 outlets that retail food, beverage and tobacco (Beijing Statistics Bureau, 2004). As shown in Table 7.1, the amount of sheep and goat meat sold through retail markets in Beijing City between 1996 and 2003 ranged from 38,000 t in 2001 to 74,000 t in 1997. Retail markets acted as the dominant channel for sheep and goat meat marketing in all years except 2001 when more product was sold through wholesale markets.

---

3. Retail markets are known in China by various terms including rural trade (*nongmao or jimao*) markets, morning markets, free markets, wet markets, or periodic markets. For a comprehensive overview of retail markets, see Chung (2004).
4. The prefecture of Heze in Shandong has a total of 520 markets of which 509 sell a range of consumer products and 11 are dedicated food markets.

**Table 7.1.** Sheep meat supplies, sales and stocks in Beijing.

| | Local sheep meat supplies* | External sheep meat supplies** | Amount sold | | | Stocks at year end |
|---|---|---|---|---|---|---|
| | | | Total | of which | | |
| | | | | Wholesale | Retail | |
| | | | *tonnes* | | | |
| 1996 | 42,922 | 2,264 | 48,304 | 4,126 | 44,178 | 2,750 |
| 1997 | 79,603 | 9,229 | 82,487 | 8,833 | 73,654 | 5,065 |
| 1998 | 50,057 | 7,859 | 59,188 | 8,019 | 51,169 | 7,877 |
| 1999 | 65,263 | 24,470 | 108,186 | 34,498 | 71,734 | 10,587 |
| 2000 | 62,150 | 20,873 | 70,156 | 21,301 | 48,856 | 4,339 |
| 2001 | 58,971 | 19,657 | 78,115 | 40,287 | 37,829 | 4,494 |
| 2002 | 51,278 | 17,093 | 69,020 | 28,555 | 40,465 | 4,252 |
| 2003 | | | 60,723 | 15,459 | 45,264 | 1,035 |

*Includes sheep meat from slaughtered sheep raised in Beijing and the meat equivalent of live sheep exported out of Beijing.
**Sheep meat imported from other provinces along with the meat equivalent of live sheep imported to Beijing.
*Source*: Beijing Statistics Bureau (various years).

Stalls that sell sheep meat at retail markets such as those pictured in Image 7.6 are owned and operated by members of slaughter households or by independent households. Meat is usually sold fresh on the day (usually the morning) it was slaughtered, especially outside of winter months. The quality and the value of the sheep meat are low and it is difficult to discern separate cuts. At larger urban retail markets, however, a greater range and higher quality of sheep meat products is available. In these markets, consumers can purchase various cuts of chilled or frozen product or sliced sheep meat for hot pot. Some companies or their agents have established stalls at the markets to specifically market and brand sheep meat and sheep meat products.

### 7.2.2 Wholesale markets

In the transport and distribution hubs of agricultural regions and in the suburbs of large cities, wholesale markets exist for selling and buying a range of agricultural products, including sheep meat. Central government recognizes about 300 large wholesale markets throughout China. Wholesale markets in China not only serve as a trading centre for smaller retailers to source supplies but also serve buyers from hotels, restaurants, institutional dining rooms, supermarkets and even individuals.

In Beijing, there are ten main markets that wholesale sheep meat.[5] As shown in Table 7.1, the proportion of sheep and goat meat sold through the ten whole-sale markets made up a significant proportion of all retail sales. The share of wholesale markets in total sales increased from less than 10% in 1996 to over 50% in 2001 before reducing somewhat in 2003. Table 7.1 also highlights that external (non local) supplies have increased from only 5% of all supplies in 1996

---

5. In addition to these main markets, many smaller markets wholesale sheep and goat meat. Beijing has 720 markets that wholesale agricultural and livestock products (Beijing Statistics Bureau, 2004).

to 25% in 2002. Stocks of sheep meat in storage, including meat stored by the state to stabilize the market, are small relative to sales volumes.

An illustration of a relatively new wholesale market that trades sheep and goat meat is the Jinghua Golden Cow Muslim Meat and Seafood Wholesale Market located at Dahongmen in the south of Beijing. The market opened in November 2003 and comprises a trading hall of 1200 $m^2$ that houses 100 stalls. This market mainly trades frozen beef and sheep and goat meat, although poultry, aquatic products, vegetables and fruits are also exchanged.

Other markets that wholesale large amounts of sheep meat in Beijing include Baliqiao and Xinfadi, where interviews were conducted in 2004 and 2006 with stallholders and market officials to derive the figures shown in Table 7.2. Around 50% of the sheep and goat meat at the Baliqiao market and 40% of the sheep and goat meat from the Xinfadi market was sourced from neighbouring Hebei Province while 20% came from Inner Mongolia. Beijing municipality itself supplied the remainder. Sales channels for stallholders at the two markets were similar with around 33% of sheep and goat meat sold to traders selling on smaller retail markets and 33% selling to small individual traders that further butcher and distribute the meat. Supermarkets accounted for 10% of sheep and goat meat purchases at the Baliqiao market but this was not the case at the Xinfadi market. Visual observations classified the sheep and goat meat in to 'low', 'mid' and 'high' grades, and over half was classified as 'low grade'. Xinfadi – where about 50 stallholders sell about 7 t of sheep meat per day and more at Chinese New Year – collects prices for a series of sheep meat products. These include (with average prices in brackets on 25 September 2006): bone out hindquarter (Rmb17), bone out forequarter (Rmb16), penis (Rmb39), stomach/rumen (Rmb7), liver (Rmb6), bones (leg) (Rmb3), ribs/rack (Rmb11.5), roll (hot pot type) (Rmb15), soft tendons (Rmb12), chuck roll (Rmb18), foot (Rmb4), head (Rmb4), tail (Rmb13), backbone/vertebrae (Rmb5.6), flap/skirt (Rmb16), kidney (Rmb21) and whole carcass (Rmb11.5). The operations of a stallholder in another wholesale market in Hohhot City in Inner Mongolia are described in Box 7.4 and shown in Image 7.5.

**Table 7.2.** Features of the Baliqiao and Xinfadi wholesale markets in Beijing, 2004.

|                                       | Baliqiao | Xinfadi |
|---------------------------------------|----------|---------|
| **Source of sheep and goat meat**     |          |         |
| Beijing                               | 30%      | 40%     |
| Inner Mongolia                        | 20%      | 20%     |
| Hebei                                 | 50%      | 40%     |
| **Sales channels for sheep and goat meat** |     |         |
| On-sold to retail markets             | 30%      | 30%     |
| Supermarkets                          | 10%      | —       |
| Hotels and restaurants                | 10%      | 10%     |
| Institutional dining rooms            | 20%      | 30%     |
| Individuals                           | 30%      | 30%     |
| **Sheep and goat meat grades**        |          |         |
| High                                  | 10%      | 15%     |
| Middle                                | 30%      | 35%     |
| Low                                   | 60%      | 50%     |

*Source*: Authors' estimates based on market visits.

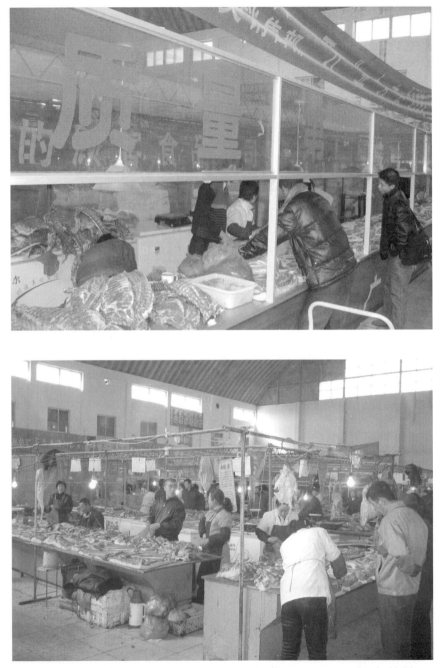

**Image 7.5(a) and 7.5(b).** Meat stallholders in the Dongwayao market in Hohhot City. The under-cover market has two areas dedicated to meat marketing and has relatively hygienic standards and facilities.

**Box 7.4.** Dongwayao food wholesale market in Hohhot City.

Wholesale markets are common throughout China and for an insight into the way they operate consider the case the Dongwayao Food Wholesale Market located in Hohhot City. This city-level market is also shown in Image 7.5. This large and relatively hygienic market is a product of the relatively strict application of regulations for meat slaughter and marketing in Hohhot, as outlined in the 'Hohhot Commercial Commodities Trading Markets Administration By-law' and the 'Hohhot Meat Trading Administration Method'. Regulations and marketing structures such as at Dongwayao occur in more progressive cities in China and provide an insight into structures that may emerge on a more widespread basis as the industry develops and as stricter hygiene regulations are promulgated and enforced.

The Dongwayao market is a large covered space that contained – among many other types of stalls – ten stalls that sold sheep meat products. Four of these had sheep meat only, three had sheep meat and other types of meat, and three had offal including that from sheep. One of the larger specialized sheep meat only stalls consisted of a 3 m long bench with room overhead for hanging and butchering. The stall holder buys about ten whole carcasses a day from the local Hohhot General Food Company. The carcasses weigh an average of 14 kg each (cleaned, bone in, fresh) and wrapped in plastic. In 2004, the stallholder paid Rmb12 per kg for the carcasses, which are delivered to the stallholder in the very early morning. The average sales price of the sheep meat is Rmb16 per kg but about half is sold 'big cuts' (such as quarter carcasses) and half is butchered into cuts. The customers of the stall are mainly restaurants, which bought specific cuts for the following prices in March 2004:

- Rmb20 per kg for eye fillet
- Rmb14 per kg for hindquarter
- Rmb14 per kg for ribs
- Rmb12.6 per kg for bone-in undifferentiated mutton
- Rmb17 per kg for bone-out undifferentiated mutton
- Rmb8 per kg for shins
- Rmb5 per kg backbone
- Rmb14 per kg for neck
- Rmb16 per kg kidney

An offal stall next to this stallholder sold:

- Rmb9 per kg for tripe
- Rmb6 per kg for lung
- Rmb11.2 per kg for cooked sheep's head

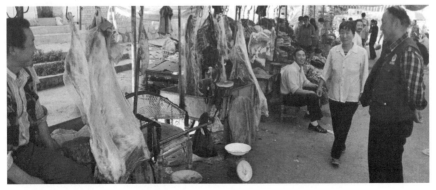

**Image 7.6.** Sheep meat stalls in an open air street market in Gansu. Sheep carcasses from a local slaughter household are hung and butchered, with a range of other food products.

### 7.2.3 Supermarkets

From a low base, the supermarket sector has grown enormously in China, as it has in many developing countries (Fritschel, 2003). In large and medium sized cities throughout China, significant volumes of sheep meat are purchased through supermarkets. The sheep meat is sourced from abattoirs, designated slaughter points and wholesale markets. In Beijing perhaps 20% of sheep meat is retailed through supermarkets, although this is much higher than most other urban areas of China.

Some supermarkets in China present sheep meat in a form that approximates Western cuts. Large refrigerated counters present packaged sheep meat in easily recognizable cuts. While not a representative example, Image 7.7 shows the display of the Yansha supermarket in Beijing which sold lamb chops, a range of delicatessen meats and smallgoods, hot pot slices, and a lamb rack (for Rmb160 per kg).

Another more representative supermarket pictured in Image 7.8 is part of the massive nationwide Hualian chain, which was also visited in Hohhot, the capital of Inner Mongolia. Partly because the city is the centre of a large sheep meat production and consumption area, the supermarket contained substantial volumes and a diverse range of sheep meat products in the supermarket. One section of the

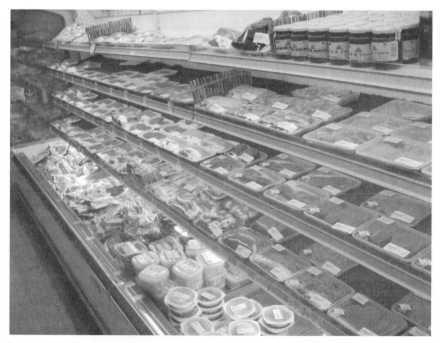

**Image 7.7.** Western style presentation of meat products in a Beijing supermarket. This supermarket targeting expatriates and wealthy Chinese has a range of meat cuts in polystyrene trays as well as a range of Chinese style processed meat products.

supermarket had a large hygienic glassed off area. At the back of the area, meat was hung in carcass form, butchered and sliced in two machines. At the front of the area was a refrigerated counter that sold a range of fresh meat. One part of the area was dedicated to selling branded beef from the Ke'erqin Fat Beef company. Next to the Ke'erqin counter was another that sold sheep meat including lamb. The source of the sheep meat was not openly advertised but further investigation revealed that it was sourced from the Hohhot General Food Company which also sold to the wholesale market mentioned in Box 7.4. Although the sheep meat was refrigerated and packaged in trays covered in cellophane in the supermarket, prices for some cuts listed in Box 7.5 were no more expensive than equivalents in the wholesale market.

Around the corner from the butchers counter were a series of refrigerated cabinets that held a range of attractively packaged pre-prepared meat products, especially sheep meat products. The Caoyuan Xingfa Company and the Yili Group had their own cabinets that sold branded products as listed in Box 7.5.

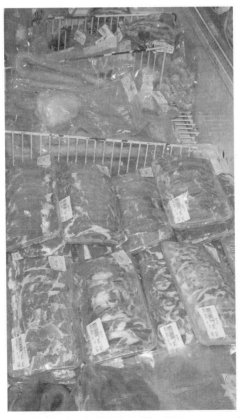

**Image 7.8.** Hualian supermarket in Hohhot City. The supermarket displays a range of hot pot sheep meat, sheep by-products and packaged processed products.

118    *China's Livestock Revolution*

---

**Box 7.5.** Prices of sheep meat products in the Hualian supermarket in Hohhot City.

---

Supermarkets often provide a diverse array of packaged, raw, semi-processed and processed products. The list below highlights some of the products and price differentiation in March 2004.

**Prices of sheep meat sourced from the Hohhot General Food Company**
- Rmb17.6 per kg for eye fillet
- Rmb17.6 per kg for hindquarter
- Rmb15 per kg for ribs
- Rmb9.2 per kg for bone-in leg meat
- Rmb17.6 per kg for bone-out leg meat
- Rmb15.6 per kg for lamb sliced for hot pot
- Rmb12.2 per kg for sheep meat mince

**Caoyuan Xingfa prepared products**
- Rmb8.2 for 300 g packet of sliced hot pot lamb
- Rmb10 for 400 g packet of sliced hot pot lamb
- Rmb7.2 for 250 g packet of beef kebabs

**Yili Group prepared products**
- Rmb9.6 for 400 g packet of sliced hot pot beef
- Rmb9.4 for 400 g packet of sliced hot pot lamb
- Rmb7.8 for 400 g packet of sliced hot pot sheep meat
- Rmb12.5 for 500 g packet of sheep meat kebabs
- Rmb6.6 for 250 g packet of sheep meat kebabs

**Yili Group packaged dumplings**
- Rmb5.8 for 400 g packet of lamb dumplings
- Rmb4.9 for 400 g packet of lamb and cabbage dumplings
- Rmb4.3 for 400 g packet lamb and carrot dumplings
- Rmb4.9 for 400 g packet lamb and celery dumplings
- Rmb5.2 for 400 g packet beef and carrot dumplings

---

Yet another part of the meat section of the Hualian supermarket in Hohhot held a range of dumplings of which sheep meat is a popular ingredient. A series of large trays sold unpackaged, machine-made dumplings from an unspecified source for Rmb11.92 per kg. These included dumplings made from mutton and onion, mutton and cabbage, mutton and carrot, mutton and shallots, and mutton and celery. The pure mutton dumplings in another tray were Rmb9 per kg. The Yili Company sold similar unpackaged dumplings made from mutton and various type of vegetable dumplings for Rmb7.2 per kg. Next to these trays was a refrigerated shelf of packaged dumplings made by the Yili Company. Box 7.5 reveals some of the price differentials that arose between these products.

Some large mutton slaughtering and processing companies have stalls (or supermarket 'sections') within supermarkets, wholesale and larger, more sophisticated retail markets. These stalls – or agents – of the companies sell branded product. This trend is highly discernible in China to the point that it dominates the way meat products are presented in many supermarkets. This can be seen as a means of differentiating product and providing quality assurance for consumers in the absence of public grading or quality assurance systems as alluded to in Chapter 5.

The evolving state of lamb and mutton marketing in China is also reflected in the increasing registration of branded products. For example, at the end of 2002, the General Administration of Commerce and Industry approved the registration of the trademark of Jingyuan Lamb, for the lamb from Jingyuan County in Gansu Province. In March 2003, after on-site and written examination by the National General Administration of Quality Supervision, Inspection and Quarantine, products of Caoyuan Xingfa Lamb (in Inner Mongolia) were successfully recommended as products of their geographic origin. Many of the examples bear out the relationship between company stalls, meat branding, higher value retail outlets and higher product quality and prices.

## 7.3 Sheep meat catering, dishes and hot pot

There are numerous dishes in China that contain sheep meat, some of which are listed in Box 7.6. Many of these dishes are derived from the traditional cuisine of Mongolian or various Muslim (including Uygur, Hui and Kazak) ethnic groups in China and account for a sizable proportion of sheep meat consumption in China. Increasing affluence and the diversification of the restaurant sector have meant that these have become very popular throughout China. In addition, there are also a significant number of dishes that are part of Han Chinese cuisine.

Sheep meat dishes are eaten at home (at levels indicated by the official statistics in Chapter 3) and in the enormous array of hotels, restaurants and institutions including dining halls. Beijing alone has approximately 60,000 dining outlets (Beijing Statistics Bureau, 2003). Sheep meat usually constitutes only a minor proportion of dishes in these outlets and are included on the menu in the interests of having a diverse and rich menu. As mentioned above, however, sheep meat – along with goat meat and beef – can be the main culinary attraction at the large number of Mongolian and Muslim food outlets.

Hot pot is arguably the most important way of eating sheep meat in urban areas of China both for China's urban restaurants as well as for in-home consumption. Hot pot has a long history but has become enormously popular in China in recent years and appears to be more than just a culinary fashion. It has established an important place in Chinese cuisine somewhere between cheap fast food outlets and expensive specialist restaurants. Various aspects of hot pot marketing and preparation are shown in Image 7.9.

Hot pot (*huo guo*) is the common name given to a method of cooking. A pot of water is placed in the middle of the table and bought to the boil. Cold, uncooked dishes of food are placed around, which customers boil in the pot. As meat is presented in very thin frozen slices, cooking time can be just a matter of seconds. The boiled food is then usually dipped in a sauce and eaten. From these basics, however, there are significant variations in the hot pot method of eating.

---

**Box 7.6.** Some dishes in China that contain sheep meat.

---

There is a wide range of dishes in China that include sheep meat as a main ingredient. Some of the dishes are:
- Leeks and lamb (*chongbao yangrou*)
- Barbequed lamb (*kao yangrou*)
- Sweet sautéed lamb (*tasimi*)
- Braised lamb with cucumbers (*weichuan yangroupian huanggua*)
- Braised lamb slices (*yangrouhu*)
- Slow cooked lamb (*qingdun yangrou*)
- Rice powder steamed lamb (*fenzheng yangrou*)
- Red cooked lamb (*hongshao yangrou*)
- Lamb in casserole (*shaguo yangrou*)
- Lamb sautéed with sauce (*jiangbao yangrou*)
- Gongbao lamb (*gongbao yangrou*)
- Sauteed shredded lamb (*chao yangrousi*)
- Vinegar-braised lamb (*culiu yangroupian*)
- Furong lamb slices (*furong yangroupian*)
- Fried lamb tenderloin (*ganzha yangliji*)
- Sautéed lamb tenderloin (*hualiu yangliji*)
- Diced lamb with brown sauce (*jiangbao yangrouding*)
- Sizzling lamb (*tieban yangrou*)
- Fried lamb (*guoshao yangrou*)
- Fried lamb rolls (*zha yang roubao*)
- Parboiled sheep tripe (*shuibao yangdu* (*huo duren*))
- Sautéed sheep tripe (*youbao yangdu*)
- Sautéed lambs stomach (*ranbao yangdu*)
- Garlic and lambs stomach (*huisuanni yangdu*)
- Sautéed 'three kinds' (lambs liver, kidney and meat) (*baosanyang*)
- Braised silver threads and garlic (*huiyingsi lansuan*)
- Assorted lamb (heart, lung, spleen, stomach, intestine and carcass)
- Braised mutton (*shoubarou*)
- Whole lamb banquet (all parts of the sheep) (*quanxi*)
- Unlike beef, lamb steaks or mutton steaks are not as popular in China, even in up-market hotels
- Xinjiang style lamb shish kebabs (*yangrouchuan*) are popular throughout China
- There are various types of soups and noodle dishes that contain mutton

---

In Mongolia fables recount Ghengis Khan's soldiers dipping meat in hot water in their helmets to improve taste and hygiene levels. In China, a traditional type of hot pot is known as *gongting* (Royal Court) which originated in Beijing and was eaten by members of the emperor's inner circle for hundreds of years. Hot pot is closely related to forms of eating like *mala huoguo* (from Sichuan), steam boat (Southeast Asia) and *shabu shabu* (in Japan). In all cases, the main types of meat used for hot pot is sheep meat, goat meat and beef. Sheep and goat meat for hot pot is known as *shuanyangrou* and beef is known as *shuanniurou*. These terms have also become synonymous with the term hot pot. There are further variations in the style of cooking hot pot:

- Pots can be made of copper (the most traditional in Beijing), clay (in Guangxi), porcelain, and even glass. *Malahuo* from Sichuan has a chimney in the middle.

- The pot can be heated with charcoal, gas, electricity, or paraffin.
- The liquid in the pot is mainly water, but can include a range of oils, herbs, spices and can, for example, be chicken flavoured, seafood flavoured or sour. The pots are sometimes divided into two or four segments which contain different types of ingredients and degrees of hot spices. In a form of hot pot popular in the south called *ganguo* (dry pot), food is cooked in beer.
- There are also a large number of different sauces that the food is dipped in after boiling. The main sauce is sesame, but there are often several others. In the south, salt is the main and sometimes only condiment.
- Variations also exist in the foods eaten. Very thinly sliced sheep meat and beef is the base of the meal and is usually accompanied by vegetables, mushrooms, tofu and noodles. Seafood (shrimps) and offal are also common, as is dog meat in the south.
- In some hot pot restaurants (including the large Xiaofeiyang chain) there has been a move toward each customer having their own individual pot of boiling water, mainly as a means of alleviating hygiene concerns in the wake of the SARS outbreak in 2003.

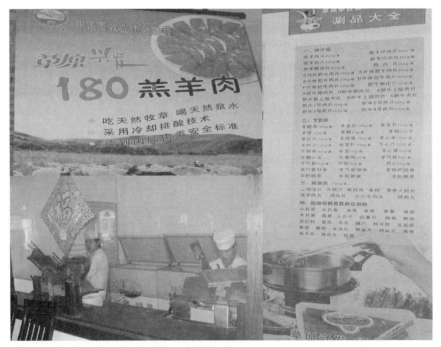

**Image 7.9.** Hot pot marketing and preparation. The top left of the collage shows pre-packaged sheep meat slices for hot pot from 180-day-old lambs, the bottom left shows the section in the restaurant where hot pot is sliced, while the right side lists the hot pot dishes produced by the Caoyuan Xingfa company including 22 meat dishes, 27 offal dishes, 9 special dishes and 27 vegetable dishes.

Hot pot has traditionally been and remains most popular in northern China. However, it has also become more popular in southern China with some differences in cooking methods mentioned above. The main meat for hot pot in north China is sheep meat slices, while in southern China it is goat meat. Black skinned goat meat commands a higher price than other goat meats in south China. These eating habits may be related more to availability and affordability because of the higher goat population in southern China, than to any intrinsic consumer preferences. Hot pot companies suggested that a lot of hot pot mutton comes from the hindquarter, which is better developed on sheep than goats. However, breed improvement programmes have sought to develop the hindquarter region of goats.

Relatedly, hot pot has traditionally been consumed predominantly in winter months which are much colder in northern China. Although a seasonal pattern still exists, in recent years hot pot restaurants have also become busy in summer months. The issue of seasonality may be borne out by mutton price variations throughout the year as reported in Chapter 3.

Hot pot is also consumed in a variety of locations. Hot pot is easily and often eaten at home and would account for a significant proportion of in-home sheep meat consumption. Households buy their ingredients (including pre-sliced sheep meat and sauces) from local markets or supermarkets. There are many individual, stand-alone hot pot restaurants that purchase their ingredients from wholesale markets. However, of increasing significance throughout China are the large chains of hot pot restaurants, which are often organized as franchises. It could be reasonably said that there would be several hot pot restaurants in every city in China, and in many cities, several in every suburb, amounting to many thousands of hot pot restaurants throughout China.

Because these chains of hot pot restaurants usually source their ingredients through central or regional headquarters, they are of enormous interest to large domestic suppliers and potentially to overseas exporters. Some of these chains – such as Caoyuan Xingfa, Xiaofeiyang and Hongwu – are totally or partly integrated from slaughter operations to food processing to franchised catering. Some of the main hot pot chains in China include:

- Caoyuan Xingfa (based in Chifeng in Inner Mongolia. A part of its large and diversified operations (overviewed in Box 7.2) is its 500 hot pot restaurants and 1000 barbeque restaurants
- Xiaofeiyang (based in Baotou in Inner Mongolia, see Box 7.7) with more than 700 restaurants
- Xiaoweiyang (based in Baotou in Inner Mongolia and has about 30 restaurants throughout China. Also produces a range of cooked mutton products and soups)
- Donglaishun/Xilaishun (based in Beijing and on the traditional Gongting style)
- Anshunxing (Beijing)
- Yangfang (Beijing)

- Jinshancheng (Chongqing)
- Huangcheng Lama (Chengdu)
- Fucheng (near Beijing, mainly beef)
- Fuhuan (near Beijing, mainly beef)
- Hongwu (Chifeng, mainly beef)

The largest hot pot chain in China – Xiaofeiyang – is profiled in Box 7.7. A Xiaofeiyang restaurant in Chifeng City in eastern Inner Mongolia employs about 70 workers. It uses about 250 kg of sheep meat per day (or 90 t per year) and 25 kg of beef per day (or 9 t per year). Another Xiaofeiyang restaurant in Zhoukou City in Henan Province, which is a major beef and cattle producing area, uses 200 kg of sheep meat and 100 kg of beef per day. The manager of the Chifeng outlet indicated that most of the sheep meat is lamb predominantly from a former General Food Company abattoir in Xilingoule League in Inner Mongolia.

**Box 7.7.** Profile of the Xiaofeiyang company.

The Xiaofeiyang Company was established in 1999 and is based in Baotou in Inner Mongolia. With a sales value of Rmb43 billion, it has grown to become one of the largest food companies in China and one of the biggest companies in Inner Mongolia.

Xiaofeiyang sources most of its sheep meat from Inner Mongolia and particularly from ten abattoirs in Xilingoule League – which is famous for the Ujumqin breed – that meet the standards of the company. It estimates that as many as 5 million sheep per year are slaughtered for Xiaofeiyang to produce 50,000 t of sheep meat. The company prefers to buy 6-month-old lambs that have a carcass weight of approximately 10 kg. They claim to pay Rmb0.2 more per kg than their main rivals – Caoyuan Xingfa – or around Rmb16 per kg bone-out end product. This meat is usually boned and prepared and packaged into rolls suitable for thin slicing.

Having purchased the sheep meat on paper at least, the Xiaofeiyang Company then on-sells the sheep meat to its franchised stores for a slightly higher price than the sheep meat it purchased (around Rmb17.06 per kg in roll form). There are 710 franchised restaurants in total, each of which is independently owned. The restaurant owners pay a service fee of Rmb500,000 per year for the use of the Xiaofeiyang brand name and for the use of company services. Dishes of 400 g of sheep meat for hot pot are purchased by the customer for between Rmb10 and Rmb30.

In addition to sheep meat, the company also use large amounts of beef, up to 130,000 t of vegetables, noodles from its own plant in Hebei and the blend for the hot pot water from its plant in Baotou. The company has also opened 22 restaurants overseas.

The company is in the process of replacing some of its sheep meat purchase channels with its own slaughter operations. The company has recently purchased and renovated two General Food Company abattoirs in Inner Mongolia (Haide and Tielong). It is also in the process of developing a new abattoir in Xilingoule with ambitious plans to increase slaughter capacity to 3 million head annually. The company has recently become more pro-active in helping (through the Animal Husbandry Bureau and local government) the pen feeding of sheep, as it is an important way of keeping up sheep supply and addressing the seasonality of its slaughter season (beyond the summer and spring months).

The meat in Xiaofeiyang restaurants is bought in packaged rolls weighing 2.5 to 4 kg. It is sliced at the restaurant (using slicing machines) and served in dishes containing 300 to 350 g of meat. Various managers thought that a woman could eat about one dish of meat and a man could eat two. That is, the hot pot style of preparation and eating facilitates higher levels of consumption of meat in one sitting than would be the case for consumption of Western style steaks.

The usual generic types of hot pot rolls contain various cuts mixed together. Within the rolls, there is some uniformity in fat cover and in the age of the sheep slaughtered (such as mutton versus lamb). However, other rolls are made from a single cut of meat and these slices stay more intact when cooking than do the mixed meat. Indeed in large restaurants, there are about 75 different types of hot pot dishes on the menu. Of the 23 meat dishes, there are ten different types of sheep meat (mainly cuts of meat but also a few types of offal) and five types of beef.

Thus the cuts used in hot pot cooking range from high value cuts like eye fillet, to hindquarter meat, to lower value rack caps and flaps. Some fat and marbling is usually required and it needs to be tender, which can be intrinsic to the carcass meat, or partially achieved by infusing fat into the muscle and by tenderizing. Purchasers buy hot pot rolls from large abattoirs and processors but stalls in wholesale markets also sell a lot of hot pot rolls which are processed, frozen and packaged by smaller plants. Many of the imports of sheep meat into China are destined for the hot pot market in the north of China because, unlike beef, there is a limited market for sheep meat in á la carte menus in Western-style restaurants and hotels.

# 8

# The revolution continues

The livestock revolution has redefined agricultural production and marketing systems, the livelihoods of participants in those systems and the diets of vast numbers of people in the developing world. Yet while the livestock revolution has ushered in enormous change, the world struggles to understand the nature of the changes and to foresee the implications. Macro-level statistics on national or regional scales can provide only partial insights.

Deeper understanding of the livestock revolution must be based on an appreciation of its complexity and multi-faceted nature. The livestock revolution has manifested itself in different ways in different countries and in different livestock industries. The revolution has been driven not just by market forces, but also by a range of other institutional and policy drivers. And it has created highly diverse and dynamic new agribusiness sectors.

The size, complexity and dynamism of the Chinese livestock sector make comprehensive, micro-level investigations of particular livestock industries such as the case study of the sheep meat industry presented in this book, the only means of gaining genuine understanding of what is happening. An investigation of the Chinese sheep meat industry illustrates well the nature of China's recent livestock revolution, having only recently undergone major development.

In the discussion of market policy and agribusiness developments in the previous chapters, four key issues or questions arose in relation to China's livestock revolution. Specifically, the questions are: is China's livestock revolution real or just an illusion, is it sustainable, what further changes lie ahead, and what are the implications of the revolution for the world livestock and meat sectors? This concluding chapter addresses these questions through insights gained from the detail in the body of this book.

To assist the discussion, a simplistic framework is presented in Figure 8.1 which highlights some of the factors important in addressing the four questions. For instance, whether the revolution is real or illusionary depends on factors such as the accuracy of statistics, the technical feasibility of achieving the levels reported in the statistics, and the compatibility of the apparent growth with incentives faced by different industry participants. Similarly, factors such as the comparative advantage of the Chinese industry, alignment of policy and market forces, and the environmental and social impacts of the rapid growth associated with the revolution will determine whether the revolution is sustainable.

As suggested by Figure 8.1, the four key questions are closely interconnected. For example, production-led growth in the initial stages of the revolution may generate domestic surpluses that will not be sustainable without substantial price corrections unless the surpluses can be exported, thereby creating an international impact. Greater international interaction will also become increasingly

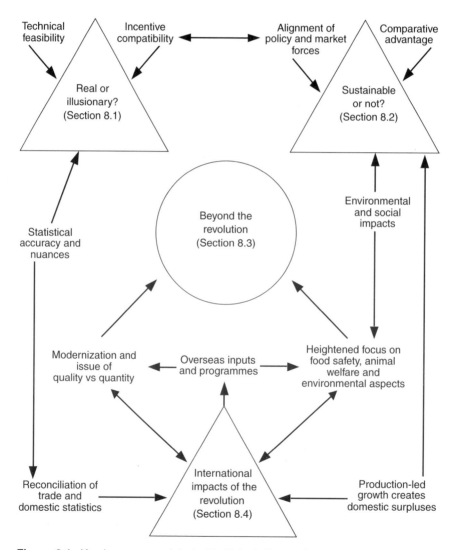

**Figure 8.1.** Key issues associated with China's livestock revolution.

important as the revolution in China moves beyond the initial stages. Further modernization and emphasis on quality rather than quantity is likely to require overseas inputs, expertise and technology, especially as more attention is focused on environmental and social matters.

## 8.1 Is the revolution real?

The extraordinary rates of growth suggested by aggregate livestock statistics coming out of China raise questions as to whether these data are believable. The validity of the official statistics is particularly important as they are used – often without verification – by a range of parties including Chinese policy makers, international agencies, trade departments, industry groups and individual traders. The analysis in this book suggests that while aggregate production and consumption statistics for the sheep meat industry must be critically analysed and treated with caution, they are not outside the bounds of reality for a number of reasons.

First, the expansion evident in the aggregate production statistics is consistent with the powerful set of market, institutional and policy forces driving industry growth. Second, the production statistics are technically feasible given common breeding and feeding regimes. Third, the statistics on items such as turnoff are likely to be more accurate for sheep than they are for other livestock types such as cattle. Fourth, there are currently relatively few constraints to throughput in producing, trading or processing sheep and sheep meat in terms of inputs, infrastructure or industry organization.

Furthermore, it appears feasible that Chinese consumers could consume all the sheep meat implied by the official production statistics. The trade balance method of deriving consumption discussed in Chapter 2 estimates that national annual consumption of sheep and goat meat in China was about 3 kg per person in 2004 while consumption in urban areas was estimated as 4.5 kg. This amount of meat could easily be consumed if meals such as hot pot, Xinjiang mutton skewers or Mongolian braised mutton – which can use 500 g of sheep meat per person per sitting – were enjoyed just once a month, or if mutton noodles and the vast array of other dishes that contain sheep meat listed in Chapter 7 were eaten weekly. Such dietary patterns are common enough in northern, western and urban parts of China to compensate for the lower consumption in southern and agricultural areas.

Although official aggregate production and consumption statistics are not unbelievable, there are good reasons to remain cautious about the rate of growth implied in the statistics. First, despite several reforms, the institution in charge of production-side data collection – the Ministry of Agriculture – is production oriented and retains incentives to over-report. This is especially the case for industries like sheep meat that have been targeted by the Chinese government for development. Second, the fragmented nature of the production, marketing and slaughtering in the sheep meat industry hinders the collection of data by a centralized authority or the verification of such data by alternative methods.

Third, major methodological problems in consumption surveys have led to the level of consumption being under-estimated. Thus it may be more accurate to derive consumption from production figures even if these are systematically inflated for the reasons mentioned above.

Given the endemic data problems, at best official aggregate livestock statistics should be treated as general indicators of trends only. In most cases the available data not only will be inaccurate but also will be presented at a level of aggregation that makes it of little value as a basis for commercial or policy decision-making. As an illustration of the commercial implications of inaccurate and highly aggregated data, abattoirs that require a continuity of supply of a specific type of livestock from a given region can not rely on official aggregate statistics on livestock numbers or turnoff. Furthermore, local officials will often exaggerate these numbers as a means of attracting investment, sometimes by a factor of 2 or 3. Although new sets of data (such as information about the scale of production) are being collected and reported publicly, the official data does not allow for sufficient differentiation between the quality and value of products. As outlined below, this differentiation will be a critical component of ongoing industry development. Thus aggregate data must be verified to the extent possible with more tailored and micro-level investigations. On a related matter, studies and policy decisions requiring more accurate macro-level data will benefit from the agricultural census planned for 2006 (and planned for reporting in 2007).

The data problems in the sheep meat industry partly reflect those in other livestock industries. For example, like sheep meat, data on beef and wool production must be collected for highly decentralized industries through bottom-up systems. However, data issues also differ between industries due to different product characteristics and systems. For example, cattle are often traded several times before slaughter. Each transaction in this case is erroneously recorded as a turnoff which is assumed in the official statistics to be a slaughtering. Dairy products are processed in more centralized facilities so milk production can be partly estimated through processing volumes. Wool is separated into three broad 'quality' categories for statistical purposes, but these categories are too broad to be of use for commercial purposes.

## 8.2 Is the revolution sustainable?

The livestock revolution in China and internationally has been widely portrayed as being driven by market forces. Although market forces can exert a large impact, the roles of institutional and policy drivers should not be overlooked, especially in China. The institutions discussed in Chapter 4 have overseen policies discussed in Chapter 5. As the sheep meat industry case study demonstrates, these policies are often taken up over-zealously at local levels. As a result, market incentives are altered for a range of industry actors, especially in the early stages of industry development.

As the sheep meat industry develops further and the market evolves and other new industries emerge, policy support for the sheep meat industry is likely to wane. This has already happened in the case of the beef industry. Policies targeted specifically at the sheep meat industry will eventually be replaced with policies targeting other industries. In addition, recently, greater emphasis is being placed on broader programmes and institutional reforms which are arguably less discriminatory between industries and more facilitative rather than interventionist with broader social objectives.

A feature of the Chinese sheep meat industry is that the policy-driven push in recent years has coincided with a strong demand-driven pull. However, some aspects of the demand-driven pull can also be argued to be short term in nature. Chinese culinary trends are notoriously volatile and consumption methods using large quantities of sheep meat – such as hot pot and Xinjiang mutton skewers – may not sustain current popularity in China unless, as discussed below, they are widely adopted by the larger rural population.

The potentially short term nature of many of the policy and market drivers of growth in the sheep meat industry means that the industry is likely to undergo rationalization within the next few years. Indeed, prices in major production areas like Xinjiang have already undergone a sharp correction and some major companies involved in the sheep breeding, contract feeding and slaughter sectors have already proven unviable. This is a signal of not only ill-conceived or poorly managed projects, but also of over supply in some sectors of the industry such as breeding and the higher value sheep meat segments of the industry.

The inevitable restructuring and rationalization of the industry is likely to be followed by a recovery and more sustainable development. Market drivers discussed in Chapter 3 – such as income growth and diversification of diet – apply strongly to sheep meat, especially as it is a relatively new part of the diversifying mainstream Chinese diet. Hot pot catering and retail markets may establish a permanent place in Chinese cuisine. And if the much heralded, but still uncertain, increase in consumption in rural areas was to take place and apply to sheep meat, growth over the longer term would be enormous. Based on figures from the trade balance method of deriving consumption in 2004, if the rural population of 757 million were to increase average annual per capita consumption of sheep and goat meat from 2 kg to 2.1 kg, an additional 230 kt of sheep and goat meat would be consumed.

The fortunate – or possibly well designed – congruence of policy-push and demand-pull forces experienced by the sheep meat industry has not always been experienced by other industries. For example, policy-push forces for the beef industry were strong in the 1990s but not matched by a concomitant surge in consumption. As a result, the industry underwent a sharp correction at the end of the 1990s. Higher value segments of the beef industry – where mechanized abattoirs and integrated feedlot facilities are most active – are still highly volatile. In the case of fine wool, for much of the late 1980s and early 1990s policy was pushing in a direction contrary to market-pull forces.

When the policies were wound back in the mid-1990s, domestic fine wool prices and production collapsed and these are unlikely to recover to previous levels. The congruence of policy-push and demand-pull forces in the sheep meat industry is perhaps most closely paralleled by the dairy industry which is also currently undergoing accelerated growth and modernization, although not without problems.

On the supply side, the long term and seemingly irreversible decline in interest in specialized fine wool production in China will provide further incentives for producers to switch into local, dual purpose or meat sheep breeds. Although the switch out of fine wool sheep can occur over a very short period, rebuilding genuine fine wool sheep flocks requires cross-breeding over many generations. The switch into local, dual purpose and meat sheep is being supported through policy, improvements in the breeding system, the extension system and various major internationally funded projects. Furthermore, these measures will increase sheep meat output even if overall sheep numbers do not increase. More specialized and market oriented production systems will increase turnoff rates, while breeding and feeding regimes oriented toward meat sheep will raise carcass weights and therefore meat output. For example, if the (low) average carcass weight for sheep and goats of 13.76 kg in 2003 was increased by just 1 kg, China would produce an extra 274 kt of sheep and goat meat. This represents nearly half the output of sheep and goat meat from major sheep meat-producing countries such as Australia or New Zealand. This technical gain could be achieved with few additional feed resources by replacing (smaller) finer wool sheep breeds with larger and hardier local, dual purpose and meat sheep breeds.

Over the longer term, questions remain about the capacity of China to increase livestock production due to feed constraints. In pastoral areas, grasslands are already grazed beyond capacity by ruminant livestock, including sheep, resulting in severely degraded grasslands. New grassland measures targeting the degradation may limit or in some areas even reduce livestock numbers in the short term. However, the Ministry of Agriculture and local governments are embarking on these grasslands measures as a means of improving grasslands, feeding practices and infrastructure to achieve precisely the opposite effect over the longer term – to increase feeding capacity and livestock numbers (see Brown *et al.*, 2007). The outcome of these initiatives has yet to be seen.

In agricultural areas, the diet of sheep and goats is based on low grade nutrition from roadside grazing, cut and carry systems and crop residues, the potential capacity of which is significantly greater than current usage.[1] Thus, the issue of whether feed supplies are a potential limit to sustained industry growth relates primarily to the availability of feed grains and fodder with a higher nutritional value. Various projects that use higher grade feed inputs to produce higher grade

---

1. China produces around 600 million t of crop residues per year. Major efforts have been made to utilize and improve the nutritional value of this feed source through programmes such as the Straw for Sheep and Goats and the Advantaged Area programmes discussed in Chapter 5.

meat sheep outputs have been implemented, as evidenced in breeding programmes, the development of feedlots and the development of integrated systems to meet specific markets. However, the viability of these systems is highly sensitive to price relativities of these higher quality feeds and sheep. If premiums for high grade meat sheep are not realized then the Chinese sheep meat industry will continue to produce low grade sheep utilizing a plentiful supply of low grade feedstuffs.

## 8.3 Beyond the revolution

Growth in China's livestock revolution can confidently be expected to continue, especially if that growth is measured in terms of quantity of production and consumption or in terms of technical indicators. Less certain, however, is the development of the industry in terms of quality or value. Although the differentiation between quality and quantity – or between industry growth and industry development – has profound importance for industry actors both within and outside China, this is an under-recognized issue.

A degree of market segmentation is occurring in the Chinese sheep meat industry but it can be difficult to discern significant premiums for quality in the industry, especially at the livestock production level. China's sheep meat industry, as is the case for other livestock industries, is dominated by the low value market segment. Generic lumps of sheep and or goat meat retail in the low value segment for between Rmb12 and Rmb16 per kg. This meat is sold predominantly through stalls in wet markets (retail or wholesale) that sell to either households for in-home consumption or to low value restaurants. The meat comes from slaughter households in nearby areas operating very low cost operations with small margins. The sheep are bought mainly through local markets at purchase prices of between Rmb6 and Rmb8 per kg liveweight. Given retail prices mentioned above and with a bone-in dressing percentage of around 45% yielding a 13 kg carcass, much of the margin for the slaughter households is in the by-products of offal, skins, bones and heads. In addition, the low selling prices and low liveweights of sheep – an average of about 30 kg – make unspecialized household sheep production a marginal activity. Indeed, if household beef cattle production is an indicator (see Longworth *et al.*, 2001, Chapter 5), meat sheep production may only appear attractive to unspecialized households if inputs such as feed and labour are undervalued or not valued at all.

Sheep meat in wholesale markets sold to mid-value restaurants or on-sold to retail markets for higher quality in-home consumption sells for Rmb16 to Rmb30 in China. However, the extremes of this range have much more to do with the region and location in which the product is sold than it does with the inherent quality characteristics of the product. Within a given region, the prices of different types of sheep meat cuts and products tend to be tightly bunched at the lower end of the mid-level price range. Sheep meat that enters this market segment can be slaughtered in designated slaughter points at modest cost or in abattoirs with added costs of about Rmb1 per kg of meat. However, households that sell better quality live sheep and lambs into this market do not appear to receive significant premiums. Prices of Rmb8 to Rmb9 per kg liveweight for sheep sold directly into large vertically integrated structures are common in pastoral areas. There are only small per kilogram price premiums for 6-month-old lambs compared with, for example, 2-year-old mutton sheep. That is, modest premiums in markets for end products become even more slender premiums at farm level. Although it is possible to see high value sheep meat (above Rmb30 per kg) in hot pot restaurants, á la carte restaurants and for some cuts in supermarkets, this is an extremely small segment of the total sheep meat market.

The international comparative advantage of the Chinese sheep meat industry may lie in the production of low value sheep meat products. However, limited international trade flows and the heterogeneity of Chinese domestic sheep meat-producing regions provide scope for a diverse domestic industry. The enthusiasm of Chinese policy makers and companies for the development of higher value markets together with the adventurous attitude to cuisine and increasing incomes of Chinese consumers will also facilitate industry segmentation. How this segmentation process develops will be of major consequence to the industry and its participants.

Because of the predominance of low value markets and low margins for small household livestock producers, various policies discussed in Chapter 5 have sought to increase quality and value in the industry. These policies tend to be interventionist in nature and emphasize physical aspects of the industry, including breeding, scale of production and large integrated processing and marketing companies or dragon heads. This supply-side approach has, if anything, crowded the lower end of mid-value market segments and put downward pressure on the price of sheep that have been bred and fed for meat purposes.

Some large dragon head enterprises have also made efforts to build mid and high value sheep meat supply chains by coordinating with local areas to produce the specified type of sheep, by introducing quality assurance programmes and by marketing new products and adopting new methods to attract new customers. A priori, these company-centred systems focused on developing higher value market segments appear desirable for industry development. In practice, this potential has been curtailed by various problems. Most fundamentally, subsidized dragon head enterprises that are not viable over the longer term 'lead' contracted households into high risk production systems. There are also widespread concerns that vertically integrated structures are not underpinned by cooperative laws, strong contractual laws or effective information feedback and pricing systems.

Beyond promoting dragon head enterprises, there are other government policies and measures that could be undertaken or improved to further encourage industry development in an inclusive way. In particular, a greater range of public market support systems to grow the mid-value segment of the market may be worth considering. As many of the premiums for mid-value meat derive from consumer confidence in food safety, better coordination and enforcement of food safety regimes and hygiene standards are likely to be of benefit.

Some of the poorer households in remote areas have livestock production systems that are less intensive than those in eastern and central China and are able to meet consumer preferences for safe foods (from 'exotic' areas). Policies designed to assist these remote area producers access the mid or higher value market segments are needed.

Market segmentation may also be facilitated through the provision of a range of other public services, including industry standards, grades and information. However, care must be exercised when considering these measures. The costs of further developing market systems for the low value mass market appear difficult to justify. For the high value market segment, large enterprises seek to differentiate their products through their own enterprise-specific systems rather than utilize broader public grading systems. However, policy-initiated steps to improve the supply chain may be more feasible for the mid-value market. Importantly, the growth of, and increased access to, the mid-value market will be of benefit to a broad range of rural actors, including household producers and small traders, especially in remote rural areas.

Investigation of ways to include and integrate remote areas and small households into mid and high value market segments highlights the need to guide industry development in a way that will bring about net social benefits. In addition to the prospect that marginal rural actors may be excluded from the benefits of the livestock revolution, there are also genuine concerns about how the livestock revolution will impact on food safety and the environment. Although this book did not deal directly with these issues, it is clear that negative impacts are occurring and may become more serious but are not inevitable. Maximizing the net social impacts from the livestock revolution will require a proactive policy approach aimed at developing targeted and effective sets of measures.

## 8.4 The revolution and international markets

The Chinese livestock revolution has largely been a domestic revolution, especially when measured by international trade flows of commodities such as sheep meat. Nevertheless, as the industry becomes more sophisticated and outgrows the domestic market, China's interaction with the world livestock sector will grow. The interaction can manifest itself in a number of way including trade, investment and technical cooperation.

The dominance and growth of the low value segments in the Chinese sheep meat industry has generated surpluses that have found export markets especially in the Middle East, to which China has also resumed the export of live sheep in modest quantities. Sheep meat and live sheep exported from China to these Middle East markets will compete closely with major exporters from countries such as Australia and New Zealand.

An interesting feature of the sheep meat industry – also applicable to the offal sector – is that exporters in Australia and New Zealand can supply into the highly price-sensitive Chinese market. This is because several cuts of sheep meat – rack cap, flaps, mutton fat and a range of offal – have a limited market and fetch low prices in the home markets of the exporting countries and so can be landed and sold in China at prices below those charged by many Chinese suppliers. Although the per unit value of these products in China is low, the significant trade volumes and the low opportunity costs of those cuts on home country markets make the China trade important for those cuts. Furthermore separating these low value cuts from higher value cuts can increase the value of the latter for other export markets.

Some limited markets exist for higher value sheep meat for the Chinese catering and supermarket trade, while niche markets – such as sheep meat labelled by country of origin on hot pot menus – can be further developed. However, these higher value market segments will increasingly be filled by domestic product as China ramps up its import replacement programme and local companies seize business opportunities as they arise.

The higher value segments of the Chinese industry require genetic, management and feedstuff inputs from overseas. Imports of sheep genetic material have become significant in recent years (see Chapter 6). In order to maintain or build this market, overseas interests should conduct trade to agreed practices (including certification), ensure that the breeds and livestock suit conditions for which they are destined and that management information and training is provided so that the breeding livestock remain productive in the Chinese environment. In addition, demand for overseas feed grains and forages may increase for Chinese sheep projects targeting higher value markets, especially given the rising opportunity costs of cropland in China. Overseas companies have already begun to export modern abattoir facilities, expertise and management systems, and this market should continue to grow.

China has strong ambitions of developing higher value sheep meat production and processing systems. The growth of these segments may in the longer term saturate the relatively small domestic Chinese market and increase pressures for export of higher value product. This export trade is currently constrained by export protocols, disease status and inadequate inspection systems. However, some regional pockets and registered company-specific systems may in the longer term gain access to higher value third country markets such as Japan and Korea.

Thus, traditional sheep meat exporters such as Australia and New Zealand not only have an interest in exporting inputs (such as genetics and feedstuffs) to capitalize on the growth of higher value sheep meat industry in China, but also in promoting the consumption of higher value products in China to reduce the pressure for China to export these products. Education and training in processing and marketing activities and in cooking techniques provided by various overseas industry groups are important in this regard. There also appears to be a strong case for more international interaction and cooperation in the areas of quality assurance and food safety, market reporting, and – in the case of the mid-value market – meat grading.

## 8.5 Concluding comment

Commentators frequently make sweeping statements about the livestock revolution in China and draw generalized conclusions in relation to the potential market for generic livestock products such as 'beef', 'wool', or 'sheep meat'. But the Chinese livestock sector, and especially the ruminant livestock part of the sector, is a rapidly changing and increasingly sophisticated part of the Chinese rural economy. The case study reported in this book demonstrates that the livestock revolution in China has created industries that exhibit major differences across geographic regions, production systems, marketing chains and market segments – to mention only some of the reasons why China-wide generalizations are, at best, of limited value and often extremely misleading. Both Chinese and foreign researchers, policymakers, industry leaders, commercial traders and others, seeking more than a superficial understanding of China's livestock revolution and its opportunities and challenges, will find it necessary to draw upon detailed micro-level studies such as that reported in this book.

# Bibliography

Anon. (2001) *Muslim Beef and Mutton from Ningxia Sold to Hong Kong Directly*, Supply and Demand InfoNet of China's Agro-products. Available at: http://www.agrisd.gov.cn/freecode.asp.

Australian Department of Agriculture Forestry and Fisheries (last accessed February 2006) *Red Meat Export Statistics*. Available at: http://www.daff.gov.au.

Ba, L., Qi, X.W., Wang, Y.L. and Dou, J.H. (2001) Neimenggu Niuyangrou Chanye Fazhan Yanjiu (Research on the Development of the Beef and Sheep and Goat Meat Industries in Inner Mongolia). *Neimenggu Caijing Xueyuan Xuebao (Inner Mongolia Institute of Finance and Economics Journal)* 2, 93–97.

Bai, Y.Y. (2002) Xibu Dakaifazhong Shengtai Huanjing Jianshe yu Yangyang Xietiao Fazhan (Environmental Protection in the Develop the West Programme and the Coordination with the Development of the Sheep Industry). *Xumu yu Shouyi (Animal Husbandry and Veterinary Medicine)* 34.

Bedard, B.G. and Hunt, T. (2004) The Emerging Animal Health Delivery System in the People's Republic of China. *World Organization for Animal Health, Scientific and Technical Review* 23 (1), 297–304.

Beijing Statistics Bureau (various years) *Beijing Statistics Yearbook*. China Statistical Publishing House, Beijing.

Brown, C.G., Longworth, J.W. and Waldron, S.A. (2002a) *Regionalisation and Integration in China: Lessons from the transformation of the beef industry*. Ashgate, Aldershot, UK.

Brown, C.G., Longworth, J.W. and Waldron, S.A. (2002b) Food Safety and Development of the Beef Industry in China. *Food Policy* 27 (3), 269–284.

Brown, C.G., Waldron, S.A. and Longworth, J.W. (2005) *Modernizing China's Industries: Lessons from wool and wool textiles*. Edward Elgar Publishing, Cheltenham, UK.

Brown, C.G., Waldron, S.A. and Longworth, J.W. (2007) *Sustainable Development in China's Pastoral Region: policy challenges, conflicts, synergies and process*. Edward Elgar, Cheltenham (forthcoming).

Burns, J.P. (2003) 'Downsizing' the Chinese State: Government Retrenchment in the 1990s. *The China Quarterly* 175, 623–856.

Cai, H.O., Longworth, J.W. and Barr, M.D. (1999) *The Mass Market for Beef and Beef Offal in Eastern China*. The State of Queensland, Department of Primary Industries, Brisbane, 62 pp., Information Series No. QI99023.

Central Committee of Chinese Communist Party (1998) *Decisions of Key Issues on Agriculture and Rural Work*. Internal Report.

Chen, W.D. and Chen, X.T. (2002) Xinjiang Yangyangye de Xianzhuang he Duice (the Situation and Countermeasures Toward the Current Situation in the Xinjiang Sheep and Goat Industry). *Caoshi Jiamu (Ruminant Livestock)* 4, 8–10.

China Sheep Association (no date-a) *Kexue Yangyang – Mianyang Gaoxiao Yufei Jishu (Scientific Sheep Raising — High Efficiency Sheep Fattening Techniques)*. China Sheep Association, 23 pp.

China Sheep Association (no date-b) *Kexue Yangyang – Mianyang yu Shanyang de Pinzhong (Scientific Sheep Raising: Sheep and Goat Breeds)*. China Sheep Association, 60 pp.

Chung, H. (2004) *China's Rural Market Development in the Reform Era*. Ashgate, Aldershot, UK.

Delgado, C., Rosegrant, M., Steinfeld, H., Ehui, S. and Courbois, C. (1999) *Livestock to 2020: The next food revolution*. International Food Policy Research Institute, Washington D.C., May, Food, Agriculture and the Environment Discussion Paper No. 28.

Deng, R. and Zhang, C.G. (2005) *Study of Animal Husbandry Development in China*, China Agriculture Press, Beijing.

Editorial Board of China Agriculture Yearbook (various years) *China Agriculture Yearbook*. China Agricultural Publishing House, Beijing.

Editorial Board of the China Animal Husbandry Yearbook (various years) *China Animal Husbandry Yearbook*. China Agricultural Publishing House, Beijing.

Editorial Board on the Breeds of Domestic Animal and Poultry in China (ed.) (1986) Shanghai Scientific and Technical Publishing House, Shanghai.

Finch, B. and Longworth, J.W. (2000) *The Hong Kong Beef Market: Opportunities for Australia*. Queensland Department of Primary Industries, Brisbane. Information Series No. QI00011.

Food and Agriculture Organization *FAOSTAT Database*. Available at: http://faostat.fao.org/

Fritschel, H. (2003) Will Supermarkets Be Super for Small Farmers? *International Food Policy Research Institute Forum* 10–12.

Fuller, F., Hayes, D. and Smith, D. (2000) Reconciling Chinese meat production and consumption data. *Economic Development and Cultural Change* 49 (1), 23–43.

Gu, X.Z., Wang, H.W. and Hu, Y.X. (1998) Yangyang Zhuanyehu Jianli zhi Wojian (Opinion on the Construction of Specialized Sheep Raising Households). *Henan Xumu Shouyi (Henan Journal of Animal Husbandry and Veterinary Medicine)* 19 (1), 30–32.

Guo, T.S. (2002) The Future Challenge. In: Guo, T.S., Sanchez, M.D. and Guo, P.Y. (eds) *Animal Production Based on Crop Residues: Chinese Experiences*. Food and Agriculture Organization Animal Production and Health Paper No. 149, pp. 185–186.

Han, J.J. and An, H.M. (2002) Yangchang Shicai de Yuanyin Fenxi (Analysis of Reasons Why a Sheep Feedlot Lost Money). *Henan Xumu Shouyi (Henan Journal of Animal Husbandry and Veterinary Medicine)* 23 (7), 32.

He, S.Q. (ed.) (2002) *Zhonghua Guobao – Xiaowei Han Yang (China's National Treasure — Small Tailed Han Sheep)*. Jinin City News Publishing House, Jining.

Hua, G.F. and Ke, Z.X. (2006) 'Caoyuan Xingfa: zhiming de huangyan (Caoyuan Xingfa: fatal lies), 21 Shiji Jingji Baodao (21st Century Economic Report). July 25, 2006.

Kangda Group (2002) Jianli Shengtai Jiazhi Chanyehua, Quanmian Tuijin Rouyang Chanyehua (Construct the Connection between the Ecology and Valuable Industry, Comprehensively Promote Meat Sheep Vertical Integration). *Guowai Xumu Keji (Overseas Livestock Science and Technology)* 29 (3), 55.

Kangda Group (2003) *Fazhan Rouyang Chanye Fugu yi Fangbaiwa (Develop the Sheep Industry — Make Everyone Rich)*, China Sheep Network. Formerly on http://www. sinosheep.com.

Ke, B.S. (2001) Recent Development in the Livestock Sector in China and Changes in Livestock/Feed Relationship. In: *Agricultural and Natural Resource Economics Discussion Paper*, No. 01/2001, School of Natural and Rural Systems Management, The University of Queensland, St Lucia.

Kui, L.J. (2002) Fazhan Rouyang Shengchan, Tigao Xumuye Jingji Xiaoyi (Develop Meat Sheep Production, Increase the Economic Efficiency of Livestock). *Qinghai Xumu Shouyi Zazhi (Chinese Qinghai Journal of Animal and Veterinary Science)* 32 (1), 39–40.

Longworth, J.W. and Brown, C.G. (1995) *Agribusiness Reforms in China: The case of wool*. CAB International, Wallingford, UK.

Longworth, J.W. and Williamson, G.J. (1993) *China's Pastoral Region: sheep and wool, minority nationalities, rangeland degradation and sustainable development*. CAB International, Wallingford, UK.

Longworth, J.W., Brown, C.G. and Waldron, S.A. (2001) *Beef in China: agribusiness opportunities and challenges*. University of Queensland Press, St Lucia, Australia.

Ministry of Agriculture (2000) *China's Tenth Five Year Plan for Livestock Industries and a Ten Year Prospective*. Internal Report.

Ministry of Agriculture (2001) *Opinion of Accelerating Livestock Development*. Internal Report.

Ministry of Agriculture (2002) National scheme for the development of animal production based on crop residues. In: Guo, T.S., Sanchez, M.D. and Guo, P.Y. (eds) *Animal Production Based on Crop Residues: Chinese Experiences*. Food and Agriculture Organization Animal Production and Health Paper, pp. 191–194.

Ministry of Agriculture (2003a) *The Development Program of Advantaged Areas in Beef Cattle and Meat Sheep and Goats Production*. Available at: http://www.agri.gov.cn/ gndt/t20030527_86492.htm.

Ministry of Agriculture (2003b) *Program of Advantaged Areas in Agricultural Products*, 26 May. Available at: www.agri.gov.cn.

Ministry of Agriculture (2003c) *Report on Domestic Animal Genetic Resources in China*. China Agricultural Press, Country Report for the Preparation of the State of the World's Animal Genetic Resources for the Food and Agriculture Organization of the United Nations.

Minter Ellison (2005) *Developments in the China Food and Beverage Industry*. China Food and Beverage Briefing Paper, May 2005.

National Bureau of Statistics (various years-a) *China Customs Statistics Yearbook*. China Statistical Publishing House, Beijing.

National Bureau of Statistics (various years-b) *China Statistics Yearbook*. China Statistical Publishing House, Beijing.

National Bureau of Statistics (various years-c) *China Price and Urban Household Budget Survey Yearbook*. China Statistical Publishing House, Beijing.

National Development and Reform Commission (2002) *Guide on Foreign Company Investment in China*. Accessed 13 March 2002. Available at: http://www.ndrc.gov.cn/

National People's Congress (2005) *Animal Husbandry Law of the People's Republic of China*, December 2005.

Nin, A., Hertel, T.W., Foster, K. and Rae, A. (2004) Productivity growth, catching-up and uncertainty in China's meat trade. *Agricultural Economics* 31 (1), 1–16.

Niu, R.F. and Xia, Y. (2000) *Nongye Chanyehua Jingying De Zuzhi Fangshi he Yunxing Jizhi (Organizational Patterns and Operation Mechanism of Agricultural Vertical Integration Management)*. Beijing University Press, Beijing.

People's Daily Online (2002a) *Chinese Beef and Mutton Popular in Muslim Nations*. Accessed 22 July 2003. Available at: http://english.peopledaily.com.cn/200208/17/print20020817_101614.html.

People's Daily Online (2002b) *Egyptian, Chinese Companies Sign Meat Deal*. Accessed 22 July 2003. Available at: http://english.peopledaily.com.cn/200212/18/print20021218_108660.html.

People's Daily (2004) 82% of the Public Is Most Worried About Food Safety: Survey. *People's Daily (English Edition)*, 5 July 2004.

Price Division of the State Development and Planning Commission (various years) *National Agricultural Products Costs and Benefits Compilation*. China Price Publishing House, Beijing.

Rozelle, S., Park, A., Benziger, V. and Ren, C. (1998) Targeted poverty investments and economic growth in China. *Food Policy* 22 (3), 191–200.

Shandong Statistics Bureau (2004) *Shandong Statistics Yearbook*. China Statistical Publishing House, Beijing.

Shen, M.G., Rozelle, S. and Zhang, L.X. (2004) *Farmer's Professional Associations in Rural China: State Dominated or New State Society Partnerships?* Unpublished manuscript.

Simpson, J.R. (2003) Long Term Projections of Livestock, Meat and Feedstuffs in China: Focus on Beef Production Potential. *Proceedings of 2003 Annual Meeting of WCC-101: China as a Market and Competitor*, Portland, Oregon, 17–18 April.

Simpson, J.R., Cheng, X. and Miyazaki, A. (1994) *China's Livestock and Related Agriculture: Projections to 2025*. CAB International, Wallingford, UK.

State Council (2003) *Opinion of Accelerating Development Processing Industry of Agricultural Products*. Internal Report.

Sun, H. (2002) Shilun Ningxia Rouyang Chanye De Fazhan Fangxiang (Preliminary Discussion of the Development Orientation of Meat Sheep Industry in Ningxia). *Jiachu Shengtai (Ecology of Domestic Animals)* 23, 2.

United States Department of Agriculture (1998) *Fasonline: Statistical Revisions Significantly Alter China's Livestock Production, Supply and Demand*. United States Department of Agriculture Foreign Agricultural Service, October 231998. Available at: http://www.fas.usda.gov/dlp2/circular/1998/98-10lp/chinarv4.htm.

Waldron, S.A., Brown, C.G. and Longworth, J.W. (2003) *Rural Development in China: Insights from the Beef Industry*. Ashgate, Aldershot, UK.

Waldron, S.A., Brown, C.G. and Longworth, J.W. (2006) State Sector Reform and Agriculture in China. *The China Quarterly*, 186.

Wang, D.Q. and Zhang, P.S. (2002) Tuiguang Jiegan Yangyang, Wancheng Wuxiang Gongcheng (Extend Straw for Sheep, Complete the Five Projects Programme). *Neimenggu Zhiliang Jishu Jiandu (Inner Mongolia Quality Science and Technology Supervision)* 3, 47.

Wang, J.M., Zhou, Z.Y. and Yang, J. (2004) How Much Animal Product Do the Chinese Consume? Empirical Evidence from Household Surveys. *Australasian Agribusiness Review* 12.

Yao, J., Guo, J., Yang, B.H. and Xiao, X.S. (2002) Gansu Youzhi Rouyang Chanye Jishu Tixi Jianli de Yanjiu (Research on Establishing a Quality Sheep and Goat Meat Industry Technology System in Gansu). *Zhongguo Caoshi Dongwu (China Ruminant Livestock)* 22 (3), 37–38.

Yin, G.C. (2002) Xuexi Waidi Jingyan, Fazhan Jiangxi Niuyangye (Study the Experience of Outside Areas, Develop the Cattle and Sheep Industries of Jiangxi). *Jiangxi Xumu Shouyi Zazhi Jiangxi (Journal of Animal and Veterinary Science)* 2, 10–11.

Yu, Y.L. (2003) *The Sheep and Goat Meat Industry in 2003 and Future Development Opportunities*, 9 April. Available at: www.mdjagri.gov.cn.

Zeng, Y.Q., Wang, H. and Chu, M.X. (2000) *Xiaoweihanyang Roupin Lihua Xingzhuang ji Shiyong Pinzhi de Yanjiu (Study on the Composition and Quality of Small Tailed Han Sheep Meat)*. Available at: http://www.agri.ac.cn/agri_net/12/12-2/12-2-18/000302. html.

Zhang, C.G. (2005) Study of Key Milk Production Bases Distribution and Development. In: China Dairy Industry Association (ed.) *Developmental Strategy for China's Dairy Industry*. China Agriculture Press, Beijng, pp. 302–320.

Zhang, L.Z. and Pan, J.W. (2002) Yangrou Shichang Fenxi yu Neimenggu Rouyangye Fazhan Zhanlue (an Analysis of the Goat and Sheep Meat Market and the Development Strategy of the Inner Mongolian Meat Goat and Sheep Industry). *Nongye Jingji Wenti (Problems in Agricultural Economics)*, supplement, 17–21.

Zhang, P.S., Zhou, Y.X. and Song, C.R. (2002) Zhongyangchang Jingying Guanli yu Jingji Xioayi Fenxi Ji Tigao Jingji Xiaoyi De Cuoshi (Analysis on the Management and Economic Efficiency of Sheep Breeding Farms and Methods of Increasing Economic Efficiency). *Xuqinye (Livestock and Poultry Industry)*, 152.

Zhao, L., Cui, J. and Li, H.W. (2002) Guoneiwai Yangyang Shengchan Qushi ji Rouyang Shengchan Xianzhuang yu Fazhan Qianjing (Trends in Sheep Production inside and Outside of China and the Prospects for Development and Current Situation for Meat Sheep Production). *Liaoning Xumu Shouyi (Liaoning Livestock and Veterinary)* 3, 32–33.

Zhao, Y.Z. (1998) *Rouyang Gaoxiaoyi Shengchan Jishu (High Efficiency Production Techniques for Meat Sheep and Goats)*. China Agricultural Publishing House, Beijing.

Zhao, Y.Z. (ed.) (1999) *Yang Shengchan Xue (the Study of Sheep and Goat Production)*. China Agricultural Publishing House, Beijing.

Zhou, Z.Y. and Tian, W.M. (eds) (2005) *Grains in China: Foodgrain, Feedgrain and World Trade*. Ashgate, Aldershot, UK.

# Index

Note: page numbers in *italics* refer to figures, tables and boxes